Reprogram Your Weight

ADVANCE PRAISE

Reprogram Your Weight **gives us a well-crafted framework for how to lose weight and keep it off for the long term.** The foundation of the approach is something I created and have used with thousands of clients and taught to hundreds of hypnosis students. Erika Flint does a great job of capturing how this applies to weight loss and I'm excited for this book to reach more people because I know it will help them where other weight loss programs have failed.

- Cal Banyan, MA, Board Certified Consulting Hypnotist, Creator of 5-PATH® Hypnosis & Hypnotherapy, and author of the book, The Secret Language of Feelings.

Reprogram Your Weight **shows you how you can use hypnosis to get back to the basics when it comes to your hunger, effectively pressing the reset button on your issues with weight.** Erika's techniques can help you get to the root of your ideas about food, question the limiting beliefs you may not even know you have, and listen to your emotions to break unconscious habits. Best of all, hypnosis offers both a customized solution as well as a shortcut to that solution.

- Erin Baebler, Co-author of Moms Mean Business: A Guide to Creating a Successful Company and Happy Life as a Mom Entrepreneur

How many cookies does it take to keep you from being lonely? How many trips to the refrigerator do you make before you're no longer bored? What will it take for you to realize food can't satisfy your emotions? When you decide to live your life fulfilled rather than filled full get the help you need from *Reprogram Your Weight*. I love this approach because it's not a diet book it's THE plan to help you change your mind about food. The techniques in this book are instantly helpful to anyone who's tired of emotional eating and the whole dieting process. Reprogram Your Weight will help you get to the underlying emotional issues so you can stop thinking about food so much and finally change your relationship to food for good.

- Karen Hand-Harper Board Certified Hypnotist
and Hypnosis Instructor

Reprogram Your Weight **is a really good read for anyone who wants to lose weight.** It explains in easy to understand and read terms how hypnosis works for weight loss. There are a lot of good stories that illustrate each strategy so that it is easy to put yourself or your clients in these stories and see a positive outcome. Erika makes connections that are often overlooked in the multi-billion dollar weight loss industry but are key to not just losing weight but in keeping it off...or as I say... changing your relationship with food forever! All the strategies and knowledge in this book are within reach of most people. It is easy, very do-able, and offers readers a new perspective on living a healthy life that is no longer focused on food but instead teaches you to focus on enjoying your life and putting your wonderful self front and center.

- Laney Coulter, BCH, CPHI, NLP, Loving Kindness
Hypnosis Center for Training and Services

Kudos to Erika Flint! Her latest book interweaves simple tools you can use every day to end emotional eating. Simple and resourceful! A wonderful read for anyone wanting to get control of their eating habits once and for all.

- **Donna M. Bloom, Board Certified Hypnotist,**
Wise Mind Hypnosis, Long Island NY.

Another weight loss book? Well yes – and no. *Reprogram Your Weight* offers something beyond the typical advice to eat less and move more. Erika Flint provides practical suggestions for real changes in behavior and beliefs. And inspiring stories of people who've made those changes, transforming their weight and their lives.

- **Catherine Johns, Professional Speaker, Coach & Author**

A great read that explores how our thoughts and feelings can keep us trapped in unwanted behaviors. *Reprogram Your Weight* is a powerful approach that provides real, practical advice that leads to sustainable weight loss, whether you're hoping to lose 10 pounds or 100. It includes inspirational stories to show how almost anyone can lose weight by the power of their minds.

- **Brenda J Titus, Board Certified Hypnotist,**
Healing Path Hypnosis

This book is a "must read" for anyone really wanting to understand the process behind weight loss. Erika has hit on many major topics that explains the struggles that so many have gone through and how this can be resolved through proven methods. Not only will the weight loss client benefit from this information, the serious hypnosis practitioner, who is serious about helping their clients find the key points to success, will benefit as well.

- Marcella Hilferty, MBA, President Hypno Path Center, LLC., NGH Board Certified Hypnotist and Certified Professional Hypnosis Instructor

This is a great book. You read all kinds of weight loss books and they all say the same thing but not this one. Erika never gives up on ideas that can really be put into your life with hypnosis and an understanding of why you can have real lasting results by the change you make inside yourself. You begin looking at food and your weight issues with a new understanding and tools to work with. I have been a relationship coach for years and weight is a big issue in relationships and with one's self esteem. I have a stack of Erika's books next to my desk and hand them out knowing that this book works.

- ToiAnn Hanson, Intuitive Relation Coach

REPR♥GRAM
YOUR
WEIGHT

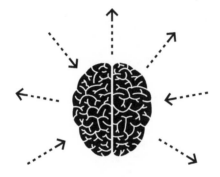

Stop Thinking about Food All the Time, Regain Control
of Your Eating, and Lose the Weight Once and for All

Erika Flint

NEW YORK

NASHVILLE • MELBOURNE • VANCOUVER

Reprogram Your Weight

Stop Thinking about Food All the Time, Regain Control of Your Eating, and Lose the Weight Once and for All

© 2017 Erika Flint

Published in New York, New York, by Morgan James Publishing in partnership with Difference Press. Morgan James is a trademark of Morgan James, LLC. www.MorganJamesPublishing.com

The Morgan James Speakers Group can bring authors to your live event. For more information or to book an event visit The Morgan James Speakers Group at www.TheMorganJamesSpeakersGroup.com.

ISBN 978-1-68350-286-9 paperback
ISBN 978-1-68350-287-6 eBook
ISBN 978-1-68350-288-3 hardcover
Library of Congress Control Number: 2016916859

Cover Design by:
Chris Treccani
www.3dogdesign.net

Interior Design by:
Chris Treccani
www.3dogdesign.net

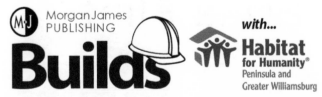

In an effort to support local communities, raise awareness and funds, Morgan James Publishing donates a percentage of all book sales for the life of each book to Habitat for Humanity Peninsula and Greater Williamsburg.

Get involved today! Visit
www.MorganJamesBuilds.com

DEDICATION

This book is dedicated to you – the reader.
To your imagination, because it will take you wherever you want to go.
And to who you are today, and the better version of yourself
tomorrow where you are light and free.

TABLE OF CONTENTS

INTRODUCTION

What Lies Behind Us and What Lies Before Us Are Tiny Matters Compared to What Lies Within Us
- Ralph Waldo Emerson

You probably *know* a lot about how to lose weight. You've likely been on many diets and plans, yet the weight always comes back - and usually with an extra 10 pounds. Knowing how to lose weight isn't enough, because if it were you'd be at your goal by now. For some reason that you wish you could figure out, you just don't seem to be able to follow through on what you need to do in order to take the weight off and keep it off for life.

And you're tired. And frustrated. And yet you haven't given up because you know if you could just lose the weight everything in your life will be better. You realize how central it is to your happiness because it really does impact every area of your life - your self-image, your job, your physical well-being and health, your mobility (or lack of it). But you're tired - you've tried so many things and are starting to wonder if maybe there's something else going on that is keeping you from being successful.

You've known other people that have lost weight, and you've also seen them wrestle with some of the same things as you do. You know you're not entirely alone with this struggle, yet your story and situation are unique, so there hasn't been any one thing that has worked for you - not without significant deprivation and effort. And not permanently.

Maybe it's always been this way, or it started when the kids came along, or after the promotion at work, or after the injury that sidelined you for a few months. Whatever it is, you feel trapped and you don't know what to do anymore - you're tired of feeling out of control, of knowing what you should be doing but not actually being able to follow through with it in a consistent way. The more you eat the more you feel out of control. And all of that leaves you feeling stuck and desperate - maybe even a bit sad or depressed. Certainly frustrated with the whole process and there are days when you want to just say "screw it" to the whole world and eat your favorite foods locked away in a quiet safe room of your home and not talk with anyone…maybe forever.

I am sorry this is happening to you. I bet you're a good person - thoughtful, compassionate, and with a kind heart. And I'm writing this book because I know of a better way… a way that will help you use something that's already inside of you to lose the weight and keep it off for good. A way that involves understanding what's *really* going on inside your heart and head that can help you lose the weight and keep it off permanently.

When you understand what your body and mind are doing that keeps the weight *on* you, you will then equally understand how to take it *off.* You will learn to use your body's natural and unique strengths to amplify your ability to lose the weight. And it doesn't include a diet or food plan. It doesn't require going to the gym or exercising for hours a day... it's something completely different, and the techniques may surprise you. And it's more than that because along the way you'll realize it's not just about losing the weight. You'll also get your life back.

I'm a hypnotherapist. I help people lose weight and make other big changes in their lives, even when everything else has failed. I hold hope in my heart for clients, even when their own hope has failed them. I help them see food for what it really is, and tap into their own power - unique for each person, that will help them eat less, move more, and lose the weight that's holding them back from the life they want to live. And all of this is done from the inside out. From the internal struggles and challenges to the application of day-to-day living in a high-speed world full of fast-food, sugar around every corner, and non-stop and conflicting diet advice.

Hypnosis works by revealing the subconscious motivations for doing things - even when we know consciously we don't want to do them. It helps us understand at a root level what the brain is doing to keep us trapped in behaviors we don't want in our life - why we can *know* what we want to do, but *feel* a completely different way.

Many aspects of modern day life contribute to weight gain and the challenge of taking the weight off - being too busy, the fact that it's easier and cheaper to buy junk food than it is to eat healthy, pressures and stress, and the social acceptance of food as entertainment.

We're also fighting biology when it comes to losing weight. Our brains don't like to feel "bad" feelings like fear or worry, and calming that part of our minds with food is not only socially acceptable, but it's very common. Donuts in the break room, and stops at the fast food restaurant on the way home are common aspects of daily living that keep people trapped in an unhealthy weight.

There's also an overwhelm of diet and health advice that creates an atmosphere of information overload. Believing we have to exercise 30 minutes a day, eat a healthy breakfast, three meals a day - or is it five small meals, and wait was I supposed to eat lunch, or fast on Fridays?

The diet advice means well, but it's often geared toward a large percentage of people - not the individual. For the individual there is one true way of knowing what you should do - and that's done by using your body's own wisdom. Tapping into that wisdom is what hypnosis gives us the power to do.

Hypnosis brings clarity to a murky landscape filled with disappointment and helps us to use our best resources for losing the weight, moving more, feeling great, and staying healthy for the rest of our lives. And the best part is that because it is part of who we naturally are, it feels effortless. It's how we are designed to operate. Once experienced, it feels as if a huge weight has been lifted. It's as if all this time we've been trying to go against the grain - yet we didn't realize it, and instead there's a way to just turn around and go in the opposite direction - going with the flow and getting a little better each and every day. And it makes all the difference.

Why Hypnosis?

In this book, I'm going to show you how hypnosis can help you with your weight loss - you'll learn how to use the mind to create healthy habits so you're not thinking about food all the time, how to regain control of eating, and how to reprogram yourself to lose weight in a way that is sustainable for the long term. By the end you'll know that everything you need to lose weight and keep it off once and for all is already inside of you.

Hypnosis Gives You Control Back

Most of my clients don't come to see me because I'm a hypnotist. They come to see me because they need help making a change in their life, and what they've tried thus far hasn't taken them where they'd like to go. They hope that hypnosis can help them.

This book is not intended to be about hypnosis - it's about how our mind and body work to form beliefs and create our experience and perceptions. Understanding how beliefs, experiences, and perceptions come about is an important aspect of our existence, and to a large extent hypnosis helps us dissect aspects of those components that aren't working for us in the way we want - but hypnosis itself is not the only way to figure these things out about ourselves. I tell my clients there are many ways to the top of the mountain - I like to use hypnosis because it provides repeatable results. And for you to have a clearer understanding of what's going on inside of you, it will help to understand a bit more about what hypnosis is and why it works.

I cannot take credit for all of the knowledge and information that I am sharing with you. The ideas regarding how hypnosis works, how the mind works and how emotions work, came from or were inspired by the work and teachings of Cal Banyan, my teacher. In this book I add my own insights and examples to what Cal teaches, and of course I focus on using that information to help you get control of your weight.

One of the most surprising aspects of hypnosis for most people is that it's a normal and natural state of mind. Without even realizing it, you've likely been in a state of hypnosis thousands of times in your life. To some extent you are in a state of hypnosis now - only it's the opposite of what you want because you're believing certain things about yourself and food that aren't even true, yet you don't realize it.

What IS Hypnosis, Really?

There are a lot of different definitions of hypnosis, but the one I like to use describes not only what hypnosis is, but also why it's helpful.

Hypnosis is a state of mind where you are highly focused and receptive to positive suggestion.

In this state of mind, you become aware of things you weren't aware of before, leading to important insights and mental clarity.

It's as if you're able to get a clearer picture of what's really been going on in your life - like finding a few "lost" puzzle pieces, that once discovered now make more sense about important aspects of your life.

These insights and clarity help you feel more secure and confident in everything you do and help align what you want with how you feel, so you can more easily set and follow through on goals you have for your life.

There are a few more details that help to clarify what's really going on inside of you that can help explain some of the out of control feelings you may be experiencing when it comes to food. I'd like you to think of your mind as having different aspects, or parts.

The Conscious Mind

The conscious mind is analytical and procedural, it's the part of your mind that solves math problems, and makes and checks things off of lists, for example. But this part of your mind is very limited - studies show it can hold onto only 7-9 pieces of information at any one time. You can think of this part of your mind as your point of focus - like a flashlight in a dark room. You can clearly see whatever you are pointing the flashlight at. That's the conscious mind.

The Subconscious Mind

The other part of your mind that's important to understand is your subconscious mind. Your subconscious mind is vast and unlimited. It's powerful - it stores everything that's ever happened to you in your entire life

And at times we are acting based on beliefs and habits that are stored in our subconscious mind without even realizing it.

Hypnosis gives us direct access to the subconscious mind so we can understand what is really going on, effectively switching on the overhead light and illuminating the entire room at once.

With hypnosis and tapping into the subconscious mind you get more information that leads to more insight. From this place you can find solutions that were once hidden, and connections are made. You have mental clarity and actually feel better inside at having the ability to understand the big picture and all the different parts.

Hypnosis gives us access to that deeper, bigger part of us that we call the subconscious mind.

Hypnosis Is Different, So Expect Different Results

The purpose of this book is to give you hope that things can be different - to let you know there's another way that works to lose weight and keep it off for good. It's likely different than anything you've tried before and that's good. Hypnosis is different and you can expect different results.

The first two chapters, *The Power of the Mind,* and *The Power of Emotions* help bring clarity to what is really going on inside of your mind and body that may be keeping you from being successful. You can think of these chapters as the overall strategy - the foundation supporting the hypnosis work. The chapters begin with an overview, then combine stories about a multitude of varying clients to demonstrate how the understanding applies to everyday living.

The next three chapters, *You're Not Lazy You're Tired, Strategies and Techniques for Reprogramming Yourself* and *Incremental Success* take a deeper look into the specific and common issues that hold people back, and also tactical approaches for how clients found unique solutions that helped them. The stories in these chapters are more specific and creative in their solutions - some of them may surprise you, and hopefully make you think in ways you haven't before about this issue that you will find helpful.

The last two chapters, *Flow*, and *See Food for What It Really Is*, are forward looking - not only about losing weight - but about how to create a new relationship with food that translates to an overall message for your life - how to live more joyfully and embrace the beauty and wonder of existence while living in a healthy, light, and free mind and body. Free from the struggle and chaos, free from the feeling of being out of control. Content, happy, and appreciative, enjoying food, but also enjoying other things in your life as well.

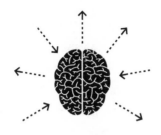

CHAPTER 1

The Power of the Mind

It's not what you look at that matters, it's what you see
- Henry David Thoreau

M ary came to me not just because she wanted to lose weight, but also because she was feeling so out of control that she wasn't enjoying any part of her life anymore. She was questioning the validity of her existence - the daily grind of going to work at a job where she wasn't appreciated, where she worked too hard to make other people money, in a relationship with her husband that was good but not great, and had been struggling to lose over 100 pounds for the better part of her adult life, at least 30 years.

Mary was a typical client in that she had tried everything on her own to lose weight that she could think of that seemed reasonable to her. There is certainly no shortage of weight loss plans and programs to be on, and she had tried all of them.

She knew how to lose weight. She'd done it plenty of times before. But she always gained it back. And she was tired of thinking about it so much. She was frustrated about trying to "solve" this problem and spending so much of her time dedicated to this one area of her life that seemed to have been her entire life focus.

Mary is good at her job, and knows how to problem solve. She's successful in practically every other area of her life, but this one thing, losing the weight, just eluded her. It always had. And she was so frustrated and tired of it that she didn't know if it was worth even trying anymore.

Mary's story had similarities to other clients' stories, but also differences. Each client has unique challenges and strengths they bring with them, and to a large extent hypnosis works by revealing what really needs to happen in order for each individual to be successful. But there are many aspects of how hypnosis works that are universal, because the truth is that hypnosis is just a word we use to describe a natural process - a way the brain can focus and become self-aware, that's been around since human existence. So it's not the hypnosis specifically that is helping - it's what the hypnosis is able to reveal paired with an understanding of how the mind and body can work together to more easily achieve desired outcomes. In this chapter we'll be looking at how our mind can hold us back from losing weight, and how hypnosis can help shift the mind away from bad habits and negative thought patterns into more positive ones.

Overwhelmed and Out of Control

"I'm *always* thinking about food and trying to lose weight", Mary said during her first session. "It works for a while, but then I get tired of it. Something always happens and gets in the way. Then I gain all the weight back, plus another 10 pounds usually. I make stupid mistakes, and I'm lazy. I just don't feel like working out. It seems like I sabotage myself. I don't know what else to do."

This type of thinking is very common for people who struggle to lose weight and keep it off - the negative self-talk, thinking they're self-sabotaging, or there's something wrong with them - and who can blame them? In most cases they've followed every plan, done everything they "thought" they were supposed to do - and it still didn't work.

What they don't realize is that there are aspects of biology and how the mind actually works at play here, and by learning more about how the mind actually works, the things that once were holding them back, can now help them be successful.

Trained to Eat Wrong

We are trained from a young age to treat food in a particular way. When we're young children we're often told to "finish all the food on your plate", or "don't you want to grow up big and strong"? Many of these well-meaning statements made by adults are actually working against our biology - because if you notice how children eat you'll see they'd often rather play than eat. They're more interested in exploring the world around them, playing with their toys and other kids, than eating if they're not actually hungry.

Then as we get older, we're taught that "breakfast is the most important meal of the day" and in many cases we're not allowed to leave home without eating a "good breakfast". Lunch is at a specific time every day, so we have to eat then or not at all. This often continues into adulthood where at work we have a certain timeframe to eat lunch, and are still eating breakfast in the morning, whether we're actually hungry or not.

We're taught that food is there to help us feel better "eat something and you'll feel better". We go out for ice cream when we win the softball game, and go out for pizza when our bunny dies. Without realizing it, our social responses to food are teaching us to emotionally eat.

The problem with all of these elements that are part of our society is that it's not actually how we as humans are designed. We have something called an appetite. Our appetite is the body's natural way to tell us when it's time to eat, or when it's time to stop eating. And we're trained out of using our appetite at a very young age by being forced to eat at specific times, or eat specific amounts of food when we're not hungry.

Compare that to other common bodily functions - like knowing when to go to the bathroom for example. Ask yourself - how do you know when it's time to go to the bathroom? Do you schedule it? Do you plan it, and think about it all day long? Probably not.

One of the best ways we can get control back when it comes to eating is to **give the job of knowing when it's time to eat and how much back to the body**, and away from the thinking process. This is about reverting back to the true power that we're born with - our bodies' own wisdom built into an important aspect of our body called our appetite, and start eating when our body tells us it's time to eat and stop when we're satisfied or full. It's called Mindful Eating, and it's possible to start using our appetite again to help us achieve the weight loss we desire. Even if you don't think you have an appetite - you may surprise yourself. Many clients have reported some trepidation when it came to using their appetite to help regulate their food intake because they say they don't actually *have* an appetite and aren't sure if they know when they're satisfied or full. And it may be true - medications and illness are two things that can impact our sense of appetite. But I always ask them to just try it - wait until they're hungry to eat and see what happens. And in every case, clients are surprised to learn they do in fact have an appetite and it can help regulate their food consumption. Mindful Eating means you use your appetite to eat when you're hungry, and stop when you're full, eating healthy food in healthy portions.

The Brain Cares How You Feel

The other element keeping people trapped in weight gain is the brain's natural tendency to turn away from pain and toward pleasure. There's plenty of scientific background on how this works, but to simplify it there are two competing parts of our brain that are always working to help keep us safe and happy.

One is the limbic system. It's an older, more primitive part of our brain. The primary focus of this part of the brain is to keep us safe. It responds to emotions and motivation, is responsible for long-term memory, and it does not like to feel unsettled or unsure because those feelings are unsafe.

However, we all know we live in a world of uncertainty, so the limbic system is often unhappy. When something happens to us that we don't like - for example, we're bored, or sad, or upset, this part of the brain feels uncomfortable, and the natural tendency is for this part of the brain to get us to do something pleasurable to feel better.

This is where many people get into trouble, because when feeling bored or stressed, food will often work as a very good distractor to take the edge off. The brain is happy - momentarily, because food provides immediate gratification. The problem is that it's also short-lived, so in order for you to actually feel better, you'll have to keep eating. This is how an entire bag of cookies disappears and how we eat more than we want, which in turn can cause us to gain weight.

The other part of the brain at work here is the prefrontal cortex. This part of the brain is the newer, executive function part of the brain responsible for long-term planning. This is the part of the brain that *knows* it's not good to eat an entire bag of cookies and doesn't *want* to eat the entire bag either.

So the problem is that with these two competing parts of our brain at play, we often feel conflicted - with part of us wanting to eat the cookies to feel better now, and part of us knowing we'll regret it later.

And the real challenge comes in because *the food actually does make us feel better.* In general, the limbic part of the brain *is actually soothed by the food.* So the truth is that the food works to help us feel better - but it's only a temporary solution - we feel better only while we're actually eating. In the long run eating for emotional reasons turns into an unhealthy habit and causes weight gain.

The reason that this is important to understand is that there is a better way. The limbic system doesn't actually need food - it just wants to feel better, and there are many other things that will make this part of the brain feel better. The problem is that food works so well in the short term that many people rely upon it exclusively - so when the time comes and we're not feeling good, we only have one response. And that's to eat something. Then we feel out of control.

The first step in any change process is awareness. And for many of my clients just understanding that this is how the brain works - the reason you reach for food when you feel bored, stressed, sad, and guilty is that there's a part of your brain that just wants you to feel better - just knowing that process is part of the way the brain naturally responds can help us make a better choice because we realize there's nothing wrong with us.

For Mary, she realized that if she just took a deep breath, and stepped outside, she could often avoid the knee-jerk response to emotional triggers in her daily life. This gave her an immediate sense of control, even if it was only part of the time at first. But slowly, over time the brain begins to rewire itself. Now, instead of just having a single option to feel better - food, there are multiple options: a walk, tea, call a friend, listen to music. And with those multiple choices comes a very important component of making change: the pause. A moment to pause, reflect, and actually *choose* the way you respond to a situation so you can get the results you want.

Traditional Methods of Weight Loss Can Actually Cause Us to Eat More

Another element of thinking that holds us back from losing weight is traditional weight loss methods. Traditional methods of weight loss often require that we become fully committed to planning, preparing, and basically thinking about food all day long. But an important principal of the mind is that *whatever we focus on grows*, and therefore if we are thinking about food all day long because we're trying to manage it, we will also increase our appetite and very likely eat more.

Controlling our food by planning what we're going to eat is an important aspect of weight loss. We need to be mindful of what we are eating, but not to the extent required by most weight loss programs. There is a place for keeping a food journal - especially if what you're doing isn't working and you believe it should. But it's not a long-term solution for most people. Most of my clients want to eat healthy and enjoy it, and also enjoy other aspects of their life as well. They actually don't want to be thinking about food the majority of their day.

And controlling how we eat by managing it can actually go against the body's natural purpose of an appetite. The body is remarkably well equipped to help us know things about ourselves - like sleep when we're tired, go to the bathroom when we feel like it, put on a coat when we're cold, and eat when we're hungry.

By controlling our food to the extent that we're not allowing our body to deliver the very important hunger signal, we're bypassing the body's own wisdom, and very often over eating, and working too hard using our brain to "guess" at when and how much we should be eating instead of allowing the body to self-regulate that important natural function of the body.

Things Hiding in Plain Sight that Keep Us from Being Successful

An important aspect of the subconscious mind is its ability to formulate beliefs about ourselves, other people, and the world around us. This is in part how we learn about the world around us, and is also part of a protective aspect of the subconscious mind.

As the subconscious mind takes in information from the outside world, things that tend to consistently happen in a particular way begin to form into beliefs. Then these beliefs can become "truths" to us - something we know to be true and don't question anymore.

In many cases these "truths" can be helpful, for example, learning that something glowing red is likely hot and can burn the skin so don't touch it is a healthy belief. It's not always true though, and over time we learn to distinguish the glowing red parts that aren't hot (like a light) from a glowing red that is hot (stove or hot coals).

But there are other beliefs that we hold about ourselves and the world around us that aren't even true. These beliefs are called Limiting Beliefs. They are based on misunderstandings and "bad data" from our past. But we've believed them for so long that they've moved into the background of awareness for us and we just know them as "true" now, and don't question their validity.

This is one area where hypnosis helps us get a new perspective to notice these Limiting Beliefs and be rid of them for good.

Dad's Good Intentions with Ice Cream Cause Big Problems Later On

Here's a story to illustrate how limiting beliefs are formed.

Sara comes home from school feeling sad and a bit disappointed. She didn't get the part she wanted in the school play.

The Dad loves his little girl, and noticing that something is wrong asks what's upsetting her. She starts crying, telling her dad that she didn't get the part she wanted and she doesn't feel good about herself.

Full of love in his heart for his little girl and only wishing to help her feel better, Dad tells her "That's OK honey, I know exactly what to do. Don't you know that ice cream *always* makes everything better?"

And with that, they have some ice cream together - her favorite treat, and she does feel better...at least for a few hours.

But the next day at school, Sara doesn't feel so well. She got a few answers wrong on her spelling test, and that old familiar bad feeling - not feeling good about herself - comes back. She wishes she were back with her Dad having ice cream.

And over time, eating ice cream to "make everything better" becomes a real problem for her as she begins turning to ice cream for all the issues in her young life. She gains weight because of it, and feels even worse about herself.

An innocent and well-intended comment by her loving father had unintended consequences, and years later the little girl is struggling with her weight and with her own self-worth and self-image - relying solely on ice cream to help her feel better.

Some of our own limiting beliefs can start in the same way - innocently, or in a moment when we didn't feel good enough or smart enough. Then over time, we notice all of the instances that support that belief. But just as with the story about the little girl - they're often not even based on the truth, because although the ice cream did make her feel better temporarily, in the end she ended up feeling worse because the ice cream caused her to gain weight.

What she didn't realize until much later was that although the ice cream tasted good in the moment - it wasn't what actually made her feel better all those times with her Dad. It was the love and support of her Dad that made her feel better. Those good feelings were erroneously attributed to the ice cream itself - instead of love from her Dad.

At a later age and through the help of a compassionate hypnotist Sara was able to separate the good feelings associated with ice cream with the love of her Dad. Now, when she feels bad she reaches out to loved ones to feel better instead.

Negative Self-Talk

Mary told me she was saying things to herself that she *knew were not helpful*. Things like "Just eat it, that's what you do" (in reference to candy in the break room at work), and "I'm stupid", "My thighs are enormous, I'll never fit in those pants", and "Why can't I ever do anything right?"

Many clients think it's normal and acceptable to talk to themselves in this way. And it may be common, but I don't think it's acceptable for the very reason that you would very likely not ever talk to anyone else in the same way - so why talk to yourself that way?

There are 3 things to understand about negative self-talk:

1. Negative self-talk is a natural way our minds prioritize things. It comes from a biological construct called a *Negativity Bias*.

Our Negativity Bias is one of the things that has saved us over the course of human history. It's our brain's ability to focus on the negative for survival. Imagine that you're running for your life - being chased by a saber tooth tiger (negative), when all of a sudden you see a beautiful shiny red apple (positive). Now you haven't seen nor eaten an apple in months, maybe years, and you'd love to stop and pick up and eat that apple, but if you did, you'd be eaten by that hungry tiger. That negativity bias just saved your life. Our negativity bias has helped humans focus on the negative to survive, so it is a natural response.

2. Negative self-talk is a bad habit that has been reinforced over time, and it can be changed.

Our brains are chemical, and we often have thoughts that are just out of habit. You are not your thoughts. Habits can be changed. Understand that your first thought is *often based in biology* - our natural Negativity Bias, so *you can throw your first thought away if you don't like it.* You get to choose your second thought. This means you get to choose whether you continue with that line of thinking or not. *On second-thought is a powerful tool reminding you that you choose the second thought.*

3. Negative self-talk is a flawed technique with positive intention.

I asked Mary if she would ever talk to a good friend or a child like that - like the way she talked to herself. "Of course not", she replied, "it's not nice or helpful". At this point, Mary began to smile because she understood how this applied to her as well.

Underneath everything we do is a positive intention, and Mary was likely using negative self-talk as a motivational technique for change, but it wasn't working. And she had been doing it for so long that she didn't realize how damaging it was. She didn't realize that whatever we focus on grows. She didn't understand that if she's focusing on the negative, she'll see more of it, and pretty soon all she'll ever see is what she does wrong, which will lead to low self-esteem and feeling bad all the time.

Instead I asked her to start treating herself like she would a good friend going through a similar situation, including speaking to herself in a more positive, uplifting way. Focusing on positive self-talk and encouraging words, emphasizing what she would say to a friend going through the same thing which is usually an approach based on kindness and compassion.

Suggesting that she focus on what she was doing right, including positive qualities and what was working, the negativity decreases naturally. But there's another really important aspect here about how the mind works. Because what we focus on grows, when we focus on what we're doing right - we'll actually see more of it day after day. As we see more of it, we'll actually do more of it as well. This is an important part of making change in our life - the ability to make small, incremental changes day after day.

Self-Sabotage

Another common issue that my weight-loss clients struggle with is self-sabotage. This is usually related to knowing what they *should* be doing, but doing the *exact opposite*. This appears as though they are sabotaging their own success.

The good news is that in most cases, this self-sabotage is merely a misunderstanding of how the mind works. Remember how the limbic system just wants to feel better now? And the prefrontal cortex wants to feel better in the long term? Self-sabotage is usually an aspect of focusing only on the now - feeling better now, and paying for it later.

I call this borrowing from tomorrow's happiness. And we do it all the time. But to be clear it is NOT self-sabotage. You are merely choosing to feel better now and alleviating the needs of one part of your brain (limbic system), instead of the needs of the other part (prefrontal cortex).

You are not purposefully hurting yourself or damaging yourself, you're basically putting a band-aid on a situation instead of fixing the deeper issue once and for all.

Insight Changes How We Think and Feel

Hypnosis gives us the power to step outside our own circumstances, see the big picture, and recognize limiting beliefs about ourselves and about our relationship to food. The amazing part of this process is that it actually changes how we feel inside.

The reality is that *we almost always do what we feel*. And the brain is making us feel things that are often based on misperceptions or things that just aren't true - giving us a feeling based on a lie, so to speak - a false feeling.

And using a technique like hypnosis can not only help us understand why we want to eat when we're not hungry, but also why we don't FEEL like doing things that in our head we know would be best for us.

This is how hypnosis can provide permanent change, because it goes to the root cause and shifts how we feel about ourselves, others, and the world around us that is based in reality.

···→ PUTTING IT ALL TOGETHER ←···

How we think about things matters - it drives our behavior and helps us make important choices about our lives. But it can also work against us, and many of our thought processes are couched in biological constructs that if we don't understand, can feel like our brain is working against us, or that there's something wrong with us.

The good news is that each of us is able to change and make good use of these biological constructs to our own advantage, and using a technique like hypnosis can help us do this faster and easier than ever before.

Mary left that first hypnosis session hopeful. She realized there's nothing wrong with her, she was just thinking about things in a way that wasn't helping her - even though she didn't realize she was doing that.

She had some bad habits of thought, and after learning how the mind works to protect us, how beliefs are formed, and how the two parts of our brain often make us feel conflicted, Mary had a better understanding of herself and why she had so much trouble in the past losing weight.

With this new information about how the mind works, Mary was able to start using her appetite to help her eat in accordance with her body's natural processes and she started losing weight right away.

She also understood why she turned to food for emotional reasons, and that she wasn't self-sabotaging - she was just trying to feel better in the moment. She came up with a better response to soothe that part of the brain, which helped her feel more in control.

She also started focusing on what she was doing right, and treating herself more compassionately and noticing things that *were* working. This helped her to feel better immediately - because her reality was more hopeful, peaceful, and happy. Even before Mary lost a single ounce, she was already feeling better about herself, her ability to lose weight and keep it off for good.

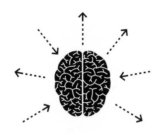

CHAPTER 2

Power of Our Emotions

We still do not know one thousandth of one percent of what nature has revealed to us.

– Albert Einstein

At any one moment in time there are over 400 ***billion*** bits of information coming into our awareness from our senses.

But we're only consciously aware of about 10 of them.

This means there are about close to 390 billion, 999 million + other bits of information that we're *not consciously aware of* that are impacting how we feel. And how we feel impacts our habits

t, like eating chips when we're stressed, or having
we're sad.

Have you ever *felt* something but couldn't put your finger on
why you felt that way? Some people call this intuition or a gut
feeling, and there could be a mystical or spiritual component to
it, but that's not what I'm referring to. I'm referring to the vast
amount of information in our awareness and the limited ability
of the conscious mind to make sense of it all in a meaningful way.

You can think of the conscious mind as a page with space
for 10 words, and the subconscious mind is a picture. A picture
is worth 1,000 words, right? Well if that's the case, then the
subconscious mind is capturing 40,000 images every second of
our life. And the conscious mind is aware of 10 words. 10 things.
Not even one full picture.

We are *very* limited by what we can consciously be aware of,
so to fix that our brain gave us emotions and feelings. In this book
I refer to emotions and feelings as the same thing, but emotions
are really the meaning applied by our subconscious mind to
any situation, and we become aware of the meaning when we
feel it in our body as a sensation - a feeling. These feelings are
a deeper knowing of the other 400+ billion bits of information
in our subconscious mind perceived from our senses plus
everything else the subconscious mind already knows based on
past experience.

Our emotions are a **powerful indicator** of what is really
going on - the big picture, and all the connected pieces. You can
think of our emotions as the result of this richer data set - and
with this additional information we can make better decisions
about ourselves and the world around us. Being in touch with
our emotions helps us stop eating for the wrong reasons, and
hypnosis helps us access our real emotions.

The Truth about Emotions

Most of us are never taught what emotions are actually for, and unlike what some people would like to believe - that emotions are fleeting, or that you shouldn't pay attention to them - they are really an indicator of what is going on in the subconscious mind. We can't always make sense of our emotions because consciously we're not always aware of what is driving them, so it can take a little time to become aware of what our emotions are trying to tell us.

Another way to think about the conscious and subconscious mind when it comes to emotions is that the conscious mind is like the tip of the iceberg. It's what you can see, and what you're aware of. The subconscious mind is what is underneath - the much larger portion of the iceberg. As discussed in the introduction, the subconscious mind has all of our memories in it - so it has a much larger database of everything that has happened to us. At times we are feeling something inside that is based on the subconscious mind, but we're not consciously aware of it yet. Many people refer to this as a "gut" feeling, and that feeling is based on a deeper understanding being driven by the subconscious mind.

The challenge is that most of us were never taught what our emotions are for, or how to address them. In many cases we were taught to ignore our emotions, and "use our head" to make decisions - when in reality our "head" is limited by what we know consciously, where our emotions are tapping into that vast body of understanding in the subconscious mind.

But years of ignoring our emotions often leaves us not understanding what they're really trying to tell us, so here's the underlying and important component: Emotions are intended to motivate us to do something - to take some action. Feeling "bad" is an indicator that something isn't right and we should do something to fix it so the "bad" feeling goes away. But because we often don't understand what the feeling is trying to tell us, we don't take action and just end up with the bad feeling instead - like feeling anxious or sad. Then we eat to distract ourselves from the bad feeling to get it to go away which causes us to over eat and usually gain weight.

One of my favorite books that goes into great detail about what our emotions and feelings are for and how to understand them is called *The Secret Language of Feelings,* by Calvin D. Banyan. I highly recommend this book and offer it to nearly all of my clients. It beautifully describes the meanings behind common feelings - like anger and boredom, and what to do about them. It also introduces the powerful concept of "Feel Bad, Distract" which is feeling bad about something, then distracting from the feeling with something else - in this case, with food.

The first thing to understand is that our emotions are worth paying attention to. They are trying to tell us something important. The emotion is often a reaction to something in our environment, and we don't *consciously* choose it. So when we find ourselves standing in the kitchen looking for something to eat, but nothing "sounds" good, that's usually an indicator that we're not actually hungry but rather bored or upset. We need to address the feeling of boredom or what's making us upset for the feeling to go away - food won't make us less bored or less upset. This is what is commonly referred to as emotionally eating - eating for an emotional reason rather than actual hunger. In this case food typically functions as a distractor - passing time so to speak, so while you're eating you're not bored or upset. But once you stop eating you will find that you're still bored or upset. This is why you may think, "hmm…. I guess it wasn't really ice cream I was hungry for - maybe I want chips instead…" and that continues until 500 calories later at which point you likely feel even worse because you still feel bored or upset, but now maybe guilty as well for eating so much.

Ignoring our emotions does not help - it does not make them go away. Trying to shove them down with food also does not help. We are often behaving based on our emotions, and the only way to address them is to understand what they're telling us, then follow through. Often when we take the time to investigate our feelings, we'll realize that what they're trying to tell us is based on false information - when that happens the "bad" feeling dissipates immediately. This happens because some of the 400+ billion bits of information that we take in through our senses are perceived incorrectly. We don't always get it right. Sometimes a look of confusion is misperceived as anger. Sometimes an email from a friend is perceived as being rude, when in fact they were just in a hurry and being very direct. If we paused for a moment to understand what we're actually feeling we may realize that our friend is not a rude person, and that they were likely just in a hurry.

However, since most of us don't know what emotions are telling us, the only conceivable option is to ignore them and hope they go away. But ignoring them almost always makes things worse.

Emotions Empower Us with a Deeper Understanding that Enables Us to See Things as They Really Are, and Live Happier Lives

Our emotions are an important part of our human makeup. They're actually an indicator of a deeper understanding - something that is usually more complex than the conscious mind in its limited ability is aware of. They help guide us to action that needs to be taken for us to be happy. This is why we often feel so conflicted and out of control - we know what we SHOULD be doing (eating a healthy dinner), but don't actually FEEL like doing it (instead we want to eat ice cream because we had a stressful day).

But our feelings are often based in misperceptions about ourselves and our surroundings, so when we learn what our emotions are telling us and where they come from we can be rid of emotions that aren't based in reality and lead much more peaceful and happy lives. But we first have to be courageous enough to feel our feelings. To know that they're there for a reason. To stop shoving them down with a cheeseburger and fries or ice cream.

Using the conscious mind only to make decisions is like buying a car and only knowing the make - not the model, not the year, and not the condition. Our emotions are complex because they include such a richer data set of everything we've experienced, but they are also capable of being understood in a simpler way. We all have this power inherent within us to understand our emotions and decode what our feelings are telling us - and hypnosis helps simplify this process for us at first - then we learn to do it on our own naturally. When we do that, it helps us feel better about ourselves and our life - and helps us do things in our life that we know we want to do - like eat healthy food that helps us feel energized, and move more.

The following stories are about clients who used hypnosis to help understand what their feelings were telling them - and in doing so they were able to discard emotional baggage that was weighing them down. Once they felt lighter emotionally, the physical weight started coming off as well.

Susan's Story: Bored, and Tired

Susan felt stuck. Every day was the same thing: wake up tired, go to work, come home exhausted, and do it all over again the next day. Even the weekends were monotonous. Days were turning into weeks, and weeks into months and years. Time was moving too fast and nothing seemed meaningful anymore. It seemed like life was passing her by, and with every passing month she felt more and more isolated. More and more alone. And she continued to gain weight.

She started her day with coffee to get her going, then it was always a race against time out the door getting everyone and everything ready and making it to work on time. But she did it. And everyone seemed happy - even Susan. She knew how to put on a happy face, and she was very good at helping other people with their problems. She was a good listener, and for some reason they seemed to come to her - telling her their issues, and so she listened politely, and helped everyone in her life with their issues as best she could.

She ate healthy food - probably just too much of it. And then there was the not so healthy food - the candy bowl at work, the donuts in the break room, and more often than not near the end of her work day, usually around 2:30 - 3 p.m. she found herself eating candy from that jar. Her plans to stop by the gym on the way home didn't sound so good anymore.

Susan was living for everyone else. She never put herself first, never felt good until everyone else in the room did also. She was so worried about everyone else that she forgot how to take care of herself and her own feelings.

Susan told me that the only time she was happy was while eating. But even that she felt guilty about, because in comparison with other people in the world - she had it pretty good. She was embarrassed to feel bad or complain about being overweight because she had a relatively happy marriage, a nice home, and a job she didn't hate.

This is how our emotions can keep us trapped: we feel bad, then we feel guilty for feeling bad which compounds the original feeling. We get stuck in a cycle of feeling bad, then worse, then eventually we're out of control and if the only thing we know to soothe ourselves is eating, well, guess what we'll be doing.

Susan would come home from work tired. She worked hard, and by the time she arrived home she was often too tired to cook something healthy. She was too tired to finish painting the guest room, or work on her garden, or go on a walk. She had given so much to her work, that the few precious hours in the evening for *her* were usually spent eating food that someone else cooked (usually take-out from a local restaurant), and watching television. She was too tired to do anything more than that.

Susan knew she needed to move more and eat less and had tried everything she could think of to make that happen. She tried going to the gym, had a treadmill at home, and had tried meal planning. But none of it ever worked long-term. She needed something that would help her be motivated to do the things she knew she needed to do.

Susan Reconnects with Her Emotions and Feels Good Again

Susan's first hypnosis session connected her with her feelings again - first the good ones. She had been unknowingly numbing herself to all her feelings for a long time because many of them were uncomfortable. In the process of blocking all the uncomfortable feelings by using food as a distractor, she lost touch with these good feelings as well. She told me later that her first session of hypnosis was life changing because she had forgotten what it felt like to feel good - to feel joy, to appreciate things in her life.

She had put food on a pedestal and was using it for everything in her life - to calm her when she was worried, to pass the time when she was bored, to fill in the gaps of an unfulfilled life. The problem is that the good feelings food provided were temporary. And she stopped doing other things in her life she enjoyed - like riding her bike and quilting.

Hypnosis gave her something nothing else could - a moment where she could gain a new perspective, a larger perspective of herself and her life and to notice what was really happening to her. She looked at her life from a bird's eye view, over the course of the last five years and the next five and realized her life seemed a bit boring - a life where food was the most important part of her day was not the life she wanted. She remembered other times in her life when she was excited. Truly excited - being fully engaged at work and using her emotions to guide her - yes, even when feeling nervous or upset at times, because those feelings helped her understand what she needed to do. They provided important insight that helped her excel at work. Then racing home after a productive work-day she looked forward to finishing a sewing project or getting on her bike.

And none of the things in her life that truly helped her feel this level of joy or excitement had to do with food - they were all experiences, adventures, and time with people she loved. Even when food was involved in the experience, it was the people and adventure that were the true elements of joy and excitement. Susan realized food had become the sole provider of happiness in her life, and that this kind of thinking was a mistake because she had so many other things in her life that brought her happiness and joy.

But the most remarkable aspect of Susan's experience was how it changed how she felt inside. When she left the hypnosis session she felt like a weight had been lifted, and she felt like her old self again - happy and excited.

Hypnosis is not alone in helping people connect with their emotions - this is how we are designed - hypnosis is just very effective at helping people tap back into that inner-knowing, that richer data set that emotions offer us, and get back in the groove, so to speak. There are other things people do to reconnect with this inner knowing, like a pilgrimage, or spending time in nature, or in peaceful meditation or prayer for example, but I like hypnosis because it's repeatable, and we get expected results.

The next week when I saw Susan for her second session, she seemed like a different person. She was happy - sparkling almost. She was so excited to share everything that happened to her that week. First she lost four pounds, and it was easier than anything else she had ever tried before - it felt effortless she reported. Part of that is because she wasn't depriving herself - she ate when she was hungry, and the other part is that she wasn't thinking about food nearly as much as she had been before. The first session of hypnosis brought her hope that things could be different, and with that hope came a sense of calm and peace; she felt more in control and found she spent her week doing other things, including cleaning out a closet that she had been meaning to clean out for over a year. She was motivated to do the things she wanted to do all along - and she felt good about cleaning it out because now she could more easily work on her sewing projects. Part of the issue she realized was that her sewing room was such a mess it was too much work to come home and work in - it was just easier to watch television. So she watched less TV as well. But what she was most amazed by was that she had gone grocery shopping, and not until she arrived at home and was unpacking her groceries did she realize that she didn't even notice the chip aisle. It's not that she saw it and had the willpower to not go down it - she didn't even see it. Something remarkable had changed inside of her - and it was that shift that helped her not notice the chips, be motivated to be active and do things she wanted to do. She felt like herself again, and she woke up in the morning excited for her day.

She ended up losing 40 pounds in a little over six months, and has since sent many clients to me. They all say the same thing - it's not the weight loss they comment on. It's her attitude; it's her joy; it's her happiness. And they hope they can get the same. And I know they can, because it's all inherently inside each of us. We just have to know how to tap back into it.

The next story I want to share is about a father who loves his family but is worried about their future, and how hypnosis revealed the secret to more security - and the healthy weight loss he desired.

Dave's Story: Dealing with Stress, Family, and Helplessness

Dave was stressed. He was a medical professional and small business owner at a local clinic, married, and father of three. He had diabetes, and an old injury that had sidelined him 10 years ago. He gained 20 pounds after the injury, and had slowly gained more weight every year since, and when he came to see me he was 35 pounds over his ideal weight.

He was worried about his health, his business, and his family if anything happened to him. On a daily basis he was working 12 hours, eating out for most of his meals, and not getting enough sleep or activity.

He felt stuck and didn't know what to do - if he worked less, he'd worry about his business and finances. Ever since the financial crash in 2008 he had been on edge, but working more didn't seem to alleviate the issue - actually it seemed to make things worse. He was spending less and less time with the family and his daughter was having a problem at school. They had been really close when she was younger, but now with him being gone so often, he didn't get to talk with her like he used to. She was about to enter a new school and he was concerned she was unhappy and struggling.

He was eating too much. He knew this, but when he was out to lunch with vendors, he forgot about that. The portions were too big when he ate out, and he'd get lost in conversation and pretty soon all of the food would be gone.

Back at the office after lunch he'd feel drained. Too much food; too much work; and he'd done the same thing again. Even after promising himself he would eat healthier this week, once he was at the restaurant and things started piling up, it was like he completely forgot about everything he was trying to do.

Dave's story is unfortunately very common. Many of us have stressful jobs that expect too much from us. Yet we are often worried about losing our financial security that a good job provides so we work harder at the expense of our health and relationships. Pretty soon we're working so hard just to keep our heads above water that we don't have time to eat healthy foods or bring a balance to our lives that would actually help us be more productive at work. We need to address the feelings of stress to understand how we can find a healthy balance to be productive at work and at home for the long run.

Dave Loses His Fear of the Future - and 14 Pounds

Hypnosis helped Dave understand that he was over eating because he was feeling helpless, but not just about his future and family but because of an old feeling of helplessness that was amplifying his current feeling state. Once he understood what was happening, he immediately felt better because he realized it didn't make sense to still be worried about things from so long ago.

The insight revealed in hypnosis that helped everything fit into place was recalling an experience he had when he was growing up. His parents were getting a divorce. He felt so helpless, and frustrated. He knew it wasn't his fault, but if they loved each other why couldn't they stay together as a family? This was the first time in his life he really felt helpless, and that was a terrible feeling. After his parents told him they were getting a divorce, they took him out for ice cream to help him feel better about the whole thing. It did help take his mind off of the situation.

The clarity that hypnosis brought helped Dave realize that he felt somewhat helpless in his life now too - the financial crisis that put his business in a tailspin was terrible. It was scary for him and his family, and he did his best to recover. He realized that ever since that time he had been eating more and more to help numb the stress of digging himself out of this financial hole. But then he realized when he was eating to reduce the stress, it was only a temporary relief, and the stress of working too much, not seeing his daughter, and gaining weight was causing a bigger issue.

He felt helpless with things in his life, but realized he was not entirely helpless. He actually had control with certain things. Like over himself. Other things that he didn't have control over he was not as worried about anymore, this peace gave him a sense of control, and it seemed like somewhat magical results because he was just not as worried about things anymore.

When Dave arrived for the third hypnosis session with a smile on his face I knew something had shifted inside of him.

"I got a great night's sleep", he said. "I've lost almost 14 pounds and my doctor lowered my blood pressure medication!" He was excited because lowering his medication was an indicator of Dave's overall health and it was a very good thing. His doctor was really surprised and happy for him as well.

Dave went on to share with me the switch that had taken place in him since he started hypnosis. The biggest change was that he felt better and more in control of his life- more at ease and less anxious and stressed which led to a lot of other little positive changes like eating less, spending more time with his family instead of work, and sleeping better.

The next story is about a woman whose situation is much different than Dave's. She wasn't stressed at all, actually she was recently retired from a high-stress job as a nurse, but the free time did not translate easily to the life she wanted - not until hypnosis helped her understand why she didn't feel like being as active as she used to be.

Amy's Story: Lonely and Never Good Enough

Amy was lonely. She knew she was lonely. She retired from her career as a nurse and tried to keep busy with volunteering and events at the church - but it wasn't enough. Those things weren't really what she wanted to be doing, but the other activities weren't an option anymore.

Her weight was keeping her from living the life she wanted, keeping her from her friends, and slowly isolating her. She could not fit in her kayak, which she was embarrassed about so she just stopped accepting invitations with her friends. And hiking hurt her knees. Camping was still an option, but she was limited to spots she could drive into, and sitting around the campfire reading wasn't nearly as much fun when everyone else was playing in the water and on the trails.

And the more she stayed at home and read, the more mundane her life became. She ate to feel better - and it helped, but as with so many things food pales in comparison to the other things in life that we really want to be doing.

And there was the issue of her brother who had died when she was younger, and she still missed him every day. It changed her life because her parents were never the same after her brother died, and she often felt both pressure to be good enough for her parents, and guilty that she was still alive and he wasn't.

Amy's story is unfortunately common. Difficult experiences create feelings inside of us - and the feelings don't just go away. Feelings are there to motivate us to do something, and unless we do what needs to be done, they'll remain. They need to be addressed.

There's an old saying "Time heals all wounds" that is absolutely false. Time does nothing to heal wounds. Time is passing, but something must happen for the wounds to heal.

And if old wounds are not addressed, they will worsen over time. Take for example, a cut finger. Time does not heal the finger - your body does, and if your body does not have the proper hemoglobin to thicken your blood, it will not heal on its own no matter how much time passes.

This has been proven time and time again in my office. Clients with experiences 50 + years ago - still in pain. Still hurting. Still angry. These issues must be addressed. You cannot change the past. But with hypnosis you can release the hurtful emotions created by past experience, just like an old wound heals over with a scar. Not perfectly back to how it was before, but so much better that you may not realize the old scar is there.

Amy Gains a New Perspective on Loss

Amy was able to see things from a new perspective that shifted how she felt about herself inside. She realized how painful it would be for her to lose a child, and could understand her parents' withdrawal from her - from life when she was younger. It didn't make it right - but she realized her parents were just people who made mistakes too. And now with this updated perspective she realized she was always good enough. That it was OK to be sad, it is the proper feeling.

And she realized something else very important. Every feeling has a purpose - to get us to do something. The good feelings basically feel good so we'll do whatever was involved to feel that way again - it's a positive feedback loop. The "bad" feelings, are just feelings we don't like. But they have a purpose too. She realized not feeling good enough and guilty were actually incorrect - but at the time they were easier than feeling the deep sadness and separation she felt from the loss of her brother. She could deal with the guilt and inadequacy, but she couldn't resolve the grief. She could see how at that time when she was younger, the guilt and inadequacy served a purpose, and that at times later in life she'd also gravitate toward feelings that were "bad" but not true either - like being mad at her husband for not taking out the garbage when she was really upset with herself for waking up late and tired - again. And now that Amy was older, she could deal with the grief. She still didn't like it, but she was better equipped to deal with it in an appropriate way than when she was a child while her parents were also suffering. She realized adults - including her parents - weren't perfect. She didn't get the help she needed to properly address her brother's death when she was little, but that was never the intention - her parents tried to help her grieve the loss of her brother, they were just ill-equipped to do it properly in their own diminished state of loss.

She allowed herself to drop into a deeper understanding of what she was really feeling. And the feeling was a sadness at the loss of her brother and a longing for something more out of life. She allowed herself to feel the loss, and realized something even more important. She loved him. That's why she was sad.

But after all this time, she also realized that being sad and focusing on the sadness wasn't really working. She wanted to do things that were working. So every time she felt sad for the loss of her brother, she flipped it around. She remembered something about him that made her smile instead. Like the other side of a coin, she flipped the sadness and allowed it to shift for her - a reminder of the time they did have together, and slowly over time the deep sadness dissipated. Along with the sadness, her anger with her parents dissolved, as did her guilt and feelings of inadequacy. She realized she had been looking at things incorrectly. But the amazing part was that all of this happened in a few short weeks. She had transformed feelings of sadness to appreciation of her own life and her ability to still do things she loved.

She easily translated this to how she was living her life. She realized decades of her "experimenting with food" for helping her to feel better never actually worked. She had been trying this experiment for 40 years of her life, and the food never helped her feel better for more than five minutes. She had a clearer understanding now why she felt so lonely and bored.

Amy started walking, and doing water aerobics. When she left the hypnosis session the first time she went to her garage, dusted off her hiking boots and went on a short hike. She found a way to make it work for her. And by spring of the next year, she was back into her kayak. She was hiking. She hasn't been camping again yet, but she's been more engaged in the things she does, spending more time with people at church. She realized that the food and television were actually boring to her - in the way she was going about her daily life. She needed something more fulfilling. She realized boring is just a feeling that reminds us to challenge ourselves - do something exciting or difficult, something that pushes us.

She's not interested in the foods she used to eat. They pale in comparison to the feeling she gets now of helping others through grief, and going kayaking and golfing with friends. And whenever she thinks of her brother, what she feels stronger than anything else is love.

····→ PUTTING IT ALL TOGETHER ←····

Our emotions are a powerful indicator of what's going on inside of us. They're the product of the 400+ billion bits of information we're not consciously aware of plus our life's past experiences - a richer data set intended on helping us understand our world and help us make decisions.

Hypnosis helps us to tap into the emotions that have been holding us back, and understand if the emotions are even valid - based in reality, or based on a misperception. Once understood, the emotions are released and we're left with insights that help guide us toward better decisions - allowing us to discard emotional baggage and feel lighter and better. We reduce emotional eating, lose weight, and begin to feel in control of our lives.

Yet emotions aren't the only area that we have misperceptions about - sometimes we have other beliefs about weight loss in general that aren't true - and if we count on them as part of our solution we will be disappointed. That's what the next chapter is all about - common misperceptions about how to lose weight.

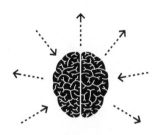

CHAPTER 3

You're Not Lazy, You're Tired

I wish I could show you when you are lonely or in darkness the astonishing light of your own being.

- Hafiz

Have you ever noticed how easy it can be to spot and help other people with their own issues, but that it can seem nearly impossible to do the same with yourself? Why is that?

One of the reasons is that as an observer you have a different perspective of a situation than a participant. When you're in a situation as a participant it's much harder to get a good handle on what's really happening because you're in the middle of it.

So many of our own issues with losing weight have to do with *mis*-perceptions about ourselves and the world around us. Yet we're too close to the situation to notice that there's anything wrong.

Wouldn't it be nice to be able to step beyond your usual frame of reference, and see your life from the observer's perspective? So you can review your own issues and hang-ups as clearly as you can others'?

That is one of the ways hypnosis can help you gain a healthy perspective on your own life, and help you more easily make changes. In hypnosis you gain the ability to shift your perspective, and take a much larger view on your life and what's been happening. It feels effortless. No more banging your head against the wall trying to "solve the problem". Hypnosis gives you the opportunity to press the pause button on your life and in a few short moments take a look at things from different angles, providing tremendous insight into your situation. And from that place of insight - free from outside distraction - you can actually shift how you feel inside. This means while in the moment - on the drive home, or sitting at your desk at work, you not only know you want to eat healthier food, but you also *feel* like it too, which means you're much more likely to do it.

Gaining a Clearer Perspective on Our Beliefs about Weight Loss

Some of the elements that keep us from losing weight are merely a belief in something that isn't even true about ourselves and the world around us - a *Limiting Belief,* as discussed in Chapter 1. Limiting Beliefs are things we believe that aren't necessarily true - only we don't know that because whether we realize it consciously or not, we've already accepted them as truth and don't question their validity -they're invisible to us.

The brain makes generalizations and assumptions about the world so we can more easily function within it. Assumptions, generalization, and educated guesses about things can help us make good decisions and protect ourselves.

But at times our beliefs about the outside world or ourselves can become over simplified or plainly incorrect - and then they become *Limiting Beliefs* because they basically keep us trapped - we base our decisions upon elements that aren't even true.

You can think of a Limiting Belief as **bad data**.

And there is a lot of "bad data" out there regarding how to lose weight and get healthy.

Some of the bad data was actually bad science - like the original 1950's research into saturated fat as causing heart disease, which has since been discredited by over 70 newer studies indicating our bodies need healthy fat. *Saturated fat does not cause heart disease* is the result concluded by one big study (The Journal Annals of Internal Medicine 2014). In the meantime, however, Americans were taught to eat a low-fat diet and consume trans-fats which many researchers indicate as the major contributing factor to the surge in weight gain in the 90's.

But other bad data is merely something we've personally gotten wrong. Like believing that we have to work out at a gym to lose weight. This type of thinking can come about because it is how we lost weight every time in the past. So we believe it is our only path to weight loss - that there isn't another way. Or believing that if we eat after 9 p.m. at night we will gain weight. Both of these assumptions are not necessarily true, but I often see clients hanging onto these ideas that keep them from losing weight.

How Bad Data Keeps Us from Losing Weight

It's pretty clear to understand how bad science can keep us from losing weight, but what about something we've just personally gotten wrong - like in the examples above with needing to go to the gym and not eating after 9 p.m. How does getting that wrong contribute to us not losing weight?

There are two ways bad data keeps us from losing weight:

1: It makes us feel bad, which leads to emotional eating

If we believe we must go to the gym to lose weight and we don't go - we feel "bad". Maybe guilty, maybe angry with ourselves. Maybe sad that we just can't seem to figure out what it takes to go to the gym. Those bad feelings then contribute to emotional eating. We feel even worse for not going to the gym, and instead eat to soothe ourselves.

2: We think there's only one way, so we don't try anything else

This truly is limiting. Take for example someone who believes their only way to lose weight - based on their past experience in the armed forces, is working out two hours a day. Since that is the only time they actually ever lost weight, they believe they must work out two hours a day to lose weight. They have incorporated this bad data into their thinking. Yet their life has changed since their time in the armed forces. They cannot feasibly work out two hours a day because they're working and taking care of a family. So instead, they feel trapped. And do nothing.

Throw Out the Bad Data

One of the truths that I want my clients to walk away with is **that they need to figure out what works for them** *now*. Not what worked for their spouse or friend. Not the latest diet or exercise trend. Not what may have worked 20 years ago before two kids and a career.

Let me ask you something - if you were doing something at work, and it just did not work, would you keep on doing it if you had any say in the matter? Most people would say absolutely not. But this is not always true with weight loss and doing what's best for ourselves. Sometimes we're so stuck in what we're doing and in the messages we're believing from our friends, family, and society, that we don't realize that what we're trying to accomplish never worked for us, and therefore we should not be doing it anymore.

Instead, we think there must be something wrong with the way we're doing it. We may even try working "harder" by putting more effort into it. And if that doesn't work then we think there may be something wrong with *us*. Somehow we have a flaw that keeps a technique from working for us when it apparently works for everyone else.

Thankfully, hypnosis allows us to uncover any flawed thinking and limiting beliefs we have about ourselves and weight loss. It gives us an opportunity to try things out for ourselves and figure out what is actually true for us, discarding the bad data. And it happens in a blink of an eye, because this type of realization while in hypnosis provides insight in a moment. Clients come into the office believing something about themselves and their own limitations, only to leave believing something completely different and usually feeling hopeful and empowered. These next stories are a few of my favorites about clients who changed their beliefs relating to how they best lose weight.

Jesse's Story: Too Tired to Be Lazy

Jessie was frustrated - "done" she said. She had stopped trying to lose the extra 30 pounds she had gained over the last 10 years. It was just too painful to keep trying and failing. She was getting more and more frustrated and disappointed.

Her problem, according to her, was that she was "lazy". She just couldn't make herself get out of bed early to go to the gym anymore like she used to. And on the way home she was more likely to run through the drive through lane of a fast food restaurant than three miles.

She believed she needed to exercise and move more, but she said was just too lazy to actually follow through on it. Her whole life she had been pretty active, and the only time she had lost weight in the past was when she was working out for an hour a day.

She thought that's what she needed to do again in order to lose the weight. It couldn't be the food she told me. She ate healthy.

I saw things entirely differently. I saw a woman who worked 10 hours a day, and spent three hours caring for her family. I saw a woman who worked so hard at her job, that by the time she came home there was 10% left on her battery. I saw a woman who didn't realize that she was actually taking in more food than her body needed - and even if it was only 100 extra calories a day, that 100 extra calories added up to around a 10-pound weight gain on average per year.

Jessie wasn't lazy. She was tired. And too focused on only one end of the equation to notice that even just a little too much food can cause unwanted weight gain.

We may want to be able to work our minds and bodies for 14 + hours a day between a job and responsibilities, but the reality is that we have human bodies that need to be replenished and that need rest.

If you are working long hours at a job, plus have other responsibilities keeping you busy, you should expect to be tired - at least a little. And a slight change in perspective can make all the difference.

Jessie believed that what worked for her in the past was the only way to move forward. This is a natural tendency for us to base our future success and plans on what worked for us in the past. It is experience-based, and there's nothing wrong with that *unless it's not actually working or feasible.* If it's not working or feasible you will need to explore other options.

A hundred years ago gyms didn't exist - not the way they do now. Why was that? Because people didn't need them. They were working hard all day. So the belief that you have to go to the gym to lose weight is not necessarily true. Actually the majority of my clients don't set foot in the gym at all. They don't like it, and the reality is that in order to do something the rest of your life it must be something you actually like. Either you like the results - like brushing your teeth every day so you can have clean teeth and gums, or you like the act itself, like walking in the park.

Consciously, Jessie knew she didn't need to go to the gym to lose weight. What I mean by that is if you asked her - Jessie do you need to go to the gym to lose weight? She'd say no. She had friends that didn't go to the gym - they hiked, walked, and kayaked and they had lost weight. *But not her.*

What Jessie didn't realize is that at a deeper level she had a limiting belief that if *she* didn't work out at the gym like she used to, she wouldn't lose weight. Going on a walk wasn't hard enough. A hike with friends wasn't enough - too much talking and fun. None of it was hard enough or painful enough to be the work necessary to lose weight.

Hypnosis enabled Jessie to take a step out of her own circumstances. It gave her the benefit of insight and honesty about her own life and the day-to-day experience. Without being so immersed in the moment itself, she was able to view her current circumstances with clarity and honesty.

Was Jessie really lazy? She was working very hard and was honestly very tired at the end of her day. Sure, it was more of a mental exhaustion, but she realized she was not lazy.

That realization made all the difference for Jessie, because when she labeled herself as lazy she bought into the idea that she just wouldn't be active anymore. She falsely believed she had an inherent flaw of being "lazy" and therefore saw it as something she'd have to use her will power to fight or overcome. Once that belief was replaced with "I'm tired", she was able to make slight adjustments into her day.

She realized she didn't need to go to the gym for 30-60 minutes a day to lose weight like she used to. Instead when she got home from work she walked for five minutes. Just 2.5 minutes out the door, and 2.5 minutes back. She could handle five minutes, and didn't dread the activity either like she did going to the gym or a long run. Over time the five-minute walk turned into 10, then 15, and eventually it became one of her favorite activities of the day - allowing her to unwind after work and fully embrace being with her family at home.

She focused on small changes in her day - she added a lunchtime walk for 10 minutes as well, and stretched during the day if she needed a break. All of these slight changes actually helped her feel energized as well.

Assumptions about ourselves and the world help us to make decisions quickly - but we can also get trapped in thinking based on bad data. Hypnosis helps provide a powerful, repeatable method of stepping beyond our conscious limitations and peering into our lives through a wider scope - with open hearts and minds. We're able to see things as they truly are.

Jessie also realized that what works for her now, as a 43-year-old mother of three, isn't going to be the same thing that worked for her when she was a 26-year-old single professional. And that's good, she realized. She didn't really want to have to work out that much. Now that her life was full of kids, a profession and a spouse, there were other things she preferred to do anyway.

Now she knows she's not lazy. But some days she does choose to rest more and relax. She recognizes the value of allowing her physical body to recover. She also knows how important it is to get up and move her physical body throughout the day - it actually gives her a quick mental break. When she returns to her desk after a short walk she has increased mental clarity and it's worth the investment of her time to take these breaks since she finds she's more effective at work.

Everything she needed to lose weight was already inside of her; she just thought she had to use it in a specific way. Now she realizes there are many ways to be successful, and as life circumstances change, she's open to change as well. Jessie lost weight consistently during our time together, and she was down eight pounds after the first month.

The next story I want to share includes a misperception related to scarcity. How a mom could unknowingly give her child a fear of poverty and hunger, and how hypnosis helped reveal the secret to removing the misperception- even when she didn't even realize it was there.

Patty: An Overweight Walking Encyclopedia of Diet Advice

Patty has never been hungry. Not really. But her mother went to bed hungry almost every night when she was a little girl and when she became a mother herself vowed to never let her children suffer the way she did.

And Patty believed her mother when she said how quickly the tides can turn. How quickly food came become sparse, and disappear. How a world war, or a natural disaster can cause a family to go hungry for weeks at a time.

It is common to adopt the fears of our parents, even if they are not true for us. They protect us from tragedy and experiences in their own life, but can also unknowingly pass down the same fear that can lead to feelings of uncertainty.

The same is true about other fears that we learn. Often when I help people with fears of spiders, snakes, and sharks, they discover that those fears were learned from their parents - but not directly. They witnessed a moment where they saw true *fear* in the eyes and faces of their parents. They weren't afraid of the spider itself, it was the look of terror it created in their mom's eyes. Whatever mom was afraid of they were afraid of now as well, even if they didn't fully understand why it was to be feared.

So Patty grew up with a fear of hunger. But she didn't realize she was afraid of it. It had been there her whole life, that underlying anxious feeling if she hadn't eaten. And she didn't know that it wasn't normal to eat all day long - "grazing" as some people called it.

For Patty, hunger was the enemy. Anytime she felt the slightest bit hungry, she became anxious and uncomfortable, so without realizing it she started a preemptive strike against her hunger and pretty much ate all day long.

But it was *healthy food* she told me! How could that make her gain weight - fruits, and vegetables, and food from her garden. Of course it was just too much for her body -even healthy food will cause us to gain weight if we eat too much of it.

And she also "knew" that she needed to eat a healthy breakfast, not eat after 9 p.m., and eat three balanced meals a day with two snacks.

But all of that "knowing" hadn't helped her to lose weight, because in reality she was actually eating all day long to keep herself from feeling uncomfortable.

Before the hypnosis session even began I asked Patty if she'd ever been hungry, or starved, as her mom had. She had not. I asked her if her mother's story was different than hers. Yes, it was, the world her mother grew up in was a different place - a place of scarcity. I asked if she believed she was in a world of scarcity now? No, there's food everywhere she replied.

What Patty didn't realize is that although her conscious mind knew there was nothing to be afraid of, at a deeper level she was still afraid, and that automated fear-based response left her feeling uncomfortable - and food always made that bad feeling go away.

Hypnosis can help by aligning what you know to be true in your conscious, thinking mind, with how you feel inside. Sometimes there's a conflict - some incongruence between what you know and what you feel. This can make daily life so challenging because you feel like you're constantly fighting yourself. And guess what, if you knew what you were fighting about, you'd likely just fix it. But the underlying issue that hypnosis helps to reveal is often something that you're aware of to some extent, but didn't realize was having this type of impact on you.

Hypnosis helped Patty release those old beliefs of fear and scarcity she had as a child, picked up from by her mother. She didn't even realize they were impacting her. She believed them then, and that belief was still in there, buried under years of mindless eating. In a state of hypnosis, Patty was able to release that old fear and that mistaken belief she learned from a well-meaning parent. Once the feeling was gone, Patty felt better. She had clarity about what had been happening, and what to do to lose weight.

But she had to prove it to herself.

She listened to her body - eating when she was hungry. Sometimes she didn't eat until 10 a.m. And she didn't like that, not at first. Just as she didn't like taking smaller portions. There was a part of her brain screaming out "that's not enough!!" but she did it anyway.

She proved it too herself. Just like so many things in our life that we thought would be one way, only to find out later they were the opposite. Patty threw away all her old thinking about food and started fresh.

Do I need to eat a healthy breakfast? She tried. Some days she was hungry early, some days not. But she loved not having to *think* about it anymore. Her brain did the planning - healthy food in the house. Then her *body* did the execution. Time to eat! Her stomach told her, and she'd eat.

Is it terrible to eat after 9 p.m.? Not if she was hungry, she realized. And not if it was healthy food. If the only thing that sounded good was junk, she knew she wasn't really hungry.

Was snacking bad? Not if she was hungry and the food was healthy.

Could she still have fun at social events while losing weight? Yes, because she started focusing on the relationships and people there instead of the food. When she did eat, she focused on portion control - just one bite, and enjoying that one bite to the fullest.

Everything she needed to lose weight was already inside of her; she just had some of her wires crossed. Some bad data. And now she's able to work for hours on her quilting and painting without thinking about food. She's lost a little weight every week, but it feels effortless because she's figured out what actually works for her. She knows she can do this for the rest of her life because she's not depriving herself, and the changes are sustainable. Now it's only a matter of time before Patty reaches her weight loss goal. But this time it will be different - she'll be able to keep it off because not only has she shifted her beliefs about herself and losing the weight, but she also knows how to spot things that aren't working for her, so she's open to making continual improvements over time.

The next story is about a different problem with food and eating - not a scarcity of food - but the pleasure of eating it. Kevin's story is about how hypnosis helped uncover something about eating pleasurable food that he wasn't aware of - and once revealed he was able to balance eating with other goals in his life like losing weight. He also learned something very important about himself.

Kevin's Story: Seeing the Hidden Price Tag for Unhealthy Food

Kevin was a foodie. He *loved* to eat. He also loved biking and drinking wine. But those three things didn't seem to go together very well because he often drank a little too much wine and didn't feel like riding, and plus he had an extra 15 pounds he had been trying to shed for the last five years. The extra weight made riding with his friends harder and he hadn't had as much fun recently for that very reason.

He came in for hypnosis because he wanted to cut back on his drinking and overeating, lose weight, and become a better cyclist.

Kevin's issue was different than Patty's: he could go for hours without food, often working through lunch and having very late dinners. But he also believed a life without good wine, cheese, and dessert wasn't one worth living. He actually had a picture in his head of himself enjoying wine, cheese, and dessert with friends after a good ride, and his bike was in the background of this picture. This was an image he created that represents his ideal life and it made him happy to think about it.

It also was part of what was causing him to over-indulge-because Kevin wasn't seeing the full picture - the true cost of what an overindulgence of high-caloric foods and alcohol was doing to his body. For Kevin, it wasn't as much a limiting belief as it was not seeing the truth about the choices he was making.

Hypnosis can help us identify and be rid of limiting beliefs as in the case of Patty and Jessie, but it can also help us see things for how they truly are. And to clarify, when I say "see things" what I mean is that people are imagining something in their mind - whether they're seeing it or just thinking about it. Not everyone actually creates pictures in their head. I'll use the word "see" for now. For some people, seeing things as they truly are means instead of seeing a bag of cookies as something that will make them happy, they see it as something that makes them happy for 10 minutes, then guilty and sad the rest of the day. It means seeing a glass of wine not as a stress reliever, but as a depressant that is actually poisonous to their body. Some clients will actually change the picture in their head - they imagine their favorite bag of cookies with a frowny face on them, or a picture of the true cost - them at their heaviest. Because that is a more accurate picture of what the cookies will do.

What if manufacturers were required to put on the outside of products what really occurred after consuming them? Would you buy a bag of chips with a picture of an overweight and unhappy person watching television on the front? What about a candy bar with a picture of an overweight and guilt-ridden person on the outside? And what about that bag of food from the drive through or take out - a picture of you feeling tired and sluggish? Next time you purchase a product, imagine the packaging as having an image of you 15 minutes after consumption. See how that changes things for you. That's truth in advertising.

Hypnosis helped give Kevin the focus and awareness to understand what he was really doing - if he liked the taste of food and wine so much, was a second or a third glass actually necessary? Was it even that good by the second glass? True wine connoisseurs spit their wine out after tasting it. What about eating the entire piece of his favorite cheesecake - was that tenth bite as good as the first?

Kevin realized the true cost of his excessive drinking - it *was* limiting his productivity at work, and it *was* keeping him from being a better cyclist. He realized if he truly loved the taste of wine, one glass would be enough. More than that, and he may have a different problem.

He also applied the law of diminishing returns to his eating. The law of diminishing returns states that the first instance of something will always be the best, subsequent instantiations will not be nearly as good. When it comes to food this means his first bite would be the best, the second would be good, but not as good as the first. His third bite would be even less enjoyable than the third.

He started seeing food for what it really was as well. The hidden price tag for eating those rich foods was keeping him from shedding his last 15 pounds, which was taking away enjoyment from his cycling - something he had been enjoying a lot longer than wine or food.

And now when Kevin looks at a bottle of wine, he actually imagines himself having one glass and being happy. His ideal image has shifted - now he pictures himself at his ideal weight laughing and enjoying one glass of wine with friends, and only a few bites of cheesecake. He's still happy, he's still enjoying his best life. But it's more balanced. And so it's easy for him to just have the one glass. He doesn't even want the second one - the second one doesn't fit into his ideal life image anymore.

···→ PUTTING IT ALL TOGETHER ←···

Jessie and Patty were both believing things about themselves and about losing weight that weren't even true. Kevin wasn't seeing the true cost of what he was putting into his body. Hypnosis helped them first identify these limiting beliefs and untruths, then shift them to a more accurate understanding of what needed to happen for them to lose weight. But it also shifted how they *felt*. Because knowing isn't enough.

With this new understanding they tried it out to see what actually worked for them - they proved it to themselves. But their work is not done. Now with this new method of making change, they're aware of how limiting beliefs can creep into their daily lives. They don't take anything for granted anymore and are constantly proving things to themselves for continual improvement.

But identifying limiting beliefs isn't the only way to make changes - sometimes we're clearly aware of what needs to be changed so it's not a limiting belief at all. Instead we're in such a habit of doing things one way that it's hard to do them any differently. The next chapter is all about habits - what are they, how are they formed, and how to change them.

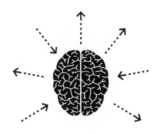

CHAPTER 4

Strategies and Techniques for Reprogramming Yourself

If you do not change direction, you may end up where you are heading.

- Lao Tzu

H ave you ever wondered how it is that you can be so good at some things - excel at work, be a great friend and parent, but really don't have it all together when it comes to figuring out how to eat healthy and lose weight? Often when we're not successful in certain areas it's because we're missing some important component - some strategy or technique that could help us.

We attempt to solve a problem with a solution that misses the mark - and for some reason we're unable to connect the dots and see that the solution isn't quite working, or that we don't actually have an improved situation. Take what happens when we eat for emotional reasons - it's merely putting a band-aid on an issue while concurrently creating new issues for us including weight gain and feelings of guilt, frustration and being out of control.

This chapter is about finding and implementing successful patterns to eat healthier, be more active, and lose weight. Some of these patterns and strategies will be brand new to you, and others will be modifications of ones you're already using - but perhaps aren't using quite right. Then we'll explore how to take these new patterns and turn them into habits - automatic programs that your brain executes without you having to think about them anymore.

Upgrading Your Habitual Programming

Do you recall what your first day of work was like? Or when you first learned to drive a car? Do you remember how overwhelming it was? And how about now - do you think about driving in the same way? We learn things over time, we have a "program" inside our subconscious mind that knows how to drive a car, and when we get into a car, that program can take over and help us drive so we don't have to consciously think about it. We can call these programs habits.

One of the most powerful ways hypnosis helps us is by illuminating the habits - programs, we already have running. Some of these programs are not helping us - like the "I'm stressed so I want to eat ice cream program". And what we want to do is replace that program with an updated version instead - one that still fits the need of the original desired outcome (reduce stress) without causing unwanted side effects (increased weight gain and possible feelings of guilt and frustration).

Why Habits Are Important to Weight Loss Success

Thus far in the book we've discussed what I call the underlying root issue - the mental and emotional components including limiting beliefs that keep us trapped. You can think of that as the foundation of the work we do. But upon the foundation there are aspects of daily life that are necessary to address as well. These aspects are the habits - good or bad, that have been built upon the foundation, and good hypnosis work is really a two-pronged approach: we address the underlying root issue (the foundation), and also look at the habitual aspects of daily life (everything built upon the foundation).

We don't want to only look at the habitual components because that merely provides a temporary fix. However, when we do both at the same time, what happens is that we positively shift how we feel inside in addition to replacing unhealthy habits for healthy sustainable ones. This works because what we are doing is shifting how we *feel*, which provides the **long-term benefit**, and then creating healthy habits that provide **immediate results**.

In neuroscience, which is the study and function of the nervous system and brain, there is an important aspect that explains why habits work called *Hebb's Law*. *Hebb's Law* states that when it comes to our brain and neurons: *whatever fires together, wires together*. It means that when we do two things together (whatever fires together), they are linked in our brain (wires together).

This is why eating and watching television can be such a problem. If you primarily eat while watching television you are training your brain to connect television and eating. Now every time you watch television you may also feel like eating - even if you're not hungry because in your brain those two components - eating and watching television, are wired together.

A Closer Look at Habits: Executable Programs and Worn Down Hiking Paths

There are two ways to think about what a habit really is. First at a high-level you can think about it as an **automatic program** running in your brain, executed without you thinking about it. But it's important to understand *how* that program is executed automatically, and *why* did it become a habit in the first place - what's happening in your brain up close?

To answer the how and why, I want you to think of a habit as a **hiking path** in your brain, that's the second way. And the more automatic it is, the more worn down the hiking path is. Imagine that as far as your brain is concerned when certain situations arise, your brain wants to choose the path of least resistance, and so it will always choose the worn-down path if there is one for any given situation. The problem is we often want to do something else - have a better choice, yet in order to do that we have to create a new path so to speak. And doing that takes effort - just as creating a brand new hiking path through the wooded forest would. But it's necessary in order to get the results we want.

For example, if your go-to response for stress is to eat ice cream, you may have linked the feeling of stress with the response of eating ice cream such that anytime you feel stress, your body will remind you to have ice cream - taking you down that old, worn out path in your brain.

In order to change this habit, in hypnosis what we do is first work on removing the cause for the underlying stress itself, but then also update your response to stress by changing that old habit to a new one - creating a new path. But just like there are ways to forge a new hiking path that are better than using your feet and a stick, there are ways to change a habit that are better than others.

The Trick to Successfully Changing a Habit

The hard part when it comes to changing a habit is that the old worn out hiking path is familiar and easy. Thankfully, when we use hypnosis to adjust the underlying issue changing a habit is already easier - because you *feel* better. But you won't feel better every moment of the day, and things like feeling tired or stressed can still make things difficult.

When we're in a low-energy state - and all I mean by that is that we're tired, or feel bad for any reason at all, the brain will automatically turn to one of these pre-established paths to solve the problem. Remember from chapter 1, the limbic system in the brain does not want to feel tired or stressed, so it will do anything to make that feeling go away.

In that low energy state, you will not have the creative resources to come up with a new choice - forge a new path for example. So you will *always* choose a pre-established path. This means you have to create a new path before you feel tired, before the end of the day. This is what I call creating a **new default response.**

This is so important! Even if you wake up in the morning and say "today is going to be the day that I have a healthy dinner" and **you're sure of it in the morning,** by the evening, you're not "feeling" like it anymore. This is because when it comes to that time in the evening, you're tired. You don't have the energy to come up with an alternative action. Basically, there's more work to be done in order to make that a healthy habit.

How to Create a New Default Response

Creating a new default response is choosing ahead of time what that new hiking path will be. But it must be selected when you have the creative energy and resources to find a new default response that truly matches both the intention and feasibility of your previous response.

Take Tina for example. She regularly came home from work stressed and went straight to the fridge which took her mind off her stressful day, but left her feeling guilty and a bit ashamed. She tried doing other things - like coming home and gardening, or going to the gym, but they didn't work.

In order for a new default response to work, it needs to match the intention of the original response: take the mind off of the stressful situation, and be as reasonably feasible (easy) as eating ice cream. Going on a walk, listening to music, going in the hot tub, or talking with a friend can all be good default responses. Gardening and going to the gym were not good default responses for Tina because although they would reduce the feeling of stress, they required a lot more work. Tina needed something that was really easy to do, and required little effort - eating ice cream doesn't take much effort does it? That's why it becomes such a powerful habit. It works (temporarily) and is easy to do.

Our bodies do need to relax. We do need moments of nothing, or no-thing. We need things that are enjoyable in our life that are as easy as eating a cookie or drinking a glass of wine but that don't have the unwanted consequences. And finding those new default responses is an extremely important aspect of being able to change old habits into new ones.

Closing the Old Hiking Path

It's common in our real life to come across detours while driving, and imagine for a moment what you would do if a real hiking path that you loved to use was permanently closed - perhaps it was too dangerous or there was a new plan for that part of the land. What would you do? You'd have to find a new way. And that's effectively what hypnosis does. It creates a new pathway in your brain that keeps the positive intention of the old, but without all of the unwanted side-effects.

The following inspirational stories are all about people who were able to change their unhealthy habits using unique and creative solutions revealed during hypnosis sessions - things they likely would never have come up with without first tapping into the clarity and self-awareness that hypnosis offers.

Drink the Tea

Lisa was 120 pounds overweight. She loved her job as a nurse but it was stressful. Long hours and long days on her feet were taking a toll on her life and her health. Her job paid well, and she had a great home in a beautiful part of town with a view of the water but she rarely had time to enjoy the view or walks on the beach.

Lisa came to me because she had tried everything she could think of to lose the weight and she saw how continuing to carry extra weight was bringing even more suffering and complications to her life as she aged.

Lisa's primary issue wasn't a lack of activity - her pedometer proved she was getting in 12k steps a day, on average. Rather it was what she was eating that was making the difference. There's a saying that helps to remind us what to focus on when losing weight "Thin in the kitchen, fit in the gym". This means in order to lose weight we need to primarily focus on what we're eating because the activity aspect of the equation is secondary. The reason is that it is so easy to over eat - we can consume 500 calories in minutes, but burning the same 500 calories takes much longer. For example, on average a person will burn 100 calories per mile walked. If you walk a 20-minute mile, it would take you one hour and forty minutes to walk off what you can eat in 10. This is why we focus on what we are eating - because we get a bigger bang for the buck so to speak. But activity is still very important, it displaces time spent watching TV and eating, and it helps us feel good inside. Both are important, but we get more out of controlling consumption (what we're eating) than expenditure (what we're burning).

Lisa ate healthy during the day and up through dinner. Her real problem was once dinner was over - that is where she would gorge on licorice, and baked goods. Lisa had grown up spending time with a loving grandmother who happened to be German and showed her love through baking and sharing cakes and pies. Lisa learned to associate love with eating those baked goods, and she was still doing it at this point in her life.

I asked Lisa to estimate how much, as a percentage, of her food she was eating after dinner, and her response was 40%. She was eating 40% of her daily calories after dinner. I asked her if she was hungry at that time, and she responded that she wasn't hungry, she just wanted to eat. It was pleasurable.

Through hypnosis we worked on her desire to eat when she wasn't hungry, and Lisa learned that when she ate those baked goods at night it was bringing up that wonderful feeling she had when she was young and spending time with her grandmother. It was enjoyable after a long day to relax, eat, and watch television. She deserved it. I agreed she deserved to relax and enjoy herself, but did she deserve to be 120 pounds overweight? Did she deserve to worry about herself, and cause additional stress to her life and body while she deserved relaxing and enjoying herself? Was it possible for her to remember those loving feelings from her grandmother without the unwanted side effect of gaining weight?

I asked Lisa if it really was the cake and pie that was so important to her when she was little, or was it the meaning she applied to those cakes and pies - the love she felt from her grandmother? It was the love she replied, and her grandmother would not want Lisa to suffer with the stress of extra weight on her body. In hypnosis Lisa was easily able to identify and separate the love from her Grandmother from the baked goods. Those two had been linked together in her mind - love and baked goods. And we were going to help Lisa unlink those two so she could feel the love from her grandmother separately from the baked goods. This was an important first step for Lisa.

Then we came up with a new default response for her - one that also met her criteria of being relaxing and enjoyable and helping her feel loved - but that didn't carry the hidden price tag of excess weight gain and feelings of worry and guilt. In the hypnosis office I made a few suggestions to Lisa, and she came up with a few of her own. I know that the clients' own suggestions are almost always better, but sometimes they feel stuck, and so I throw out a few of my own that I know have worked for other clients to see if clients respond to them in a positive way.

The one we came up with for Lisa included drinking warm tea. For Lisa, the tea provided some of the same benefits as the food - it was relaxing and enjoyable: warm, soothing, and it smelled good. But most importantly, it also reminded her of her grandmother. It became Lisa's new default response, and something she started looking forward to. The appeal at first might not have been as strong as the old habit of eating the cake or pie, but with the help of hypnosis, Lisa was able to implement this new habit of drinking tea immediately after dinner, then with the added benefit of losing five pounds the first week she was easily able to stick with it - because it was working.

One of the realizations Lisa had in hypnosis was that she had been using food as a soothing technique for almost her entire life - yet it almost never worked the way it was originally intended. I asked her if food ever actually made her feel better in these cases after she was done eating it. The answer was always no, she said. "I always feel worse because I feel guilty for eating it, then I feel ashamed, and wonder if things are ever going to be different."

So now, she has tea after dinner instead of hundreds of calories of baked goods. She's lost over 40 pounds and is still losing every week. She created the new "hiking path" for her "after dinner" program and it turned into a healthy habit in a few short weeks. But the insight didn't stop there - Lisa also realized in hypnosis about the role of baked goods in her life. She remembered something her grandmother used to say about food in general, when someone would ask her grandmother if she wanted something to eat, she always responded with "one little bite".

She'd have *one little bite* of cake, and *one little bite* of pie. Lisa realized her grandmother herself never planned nor intended on eating everything she baked - so now in addition to tea after dinner, she knew *one little bite* was a good strategy the next time she wanted to have cake or pie - and at the same time it reminded her of her grandmother without over eating.

The next story is about a woman who traded in her love of diet soda for a love of nature and riding her motorcycle, and by doing so ended up feeling a sense of accomplishment and fulfillment about herself and her own life that she had never felt before. Hypnosis helped her love herself for who she really was.

Binging on Nature

Cindy worked from home and spent most of her time outside of work taking care of the house, her yard, her aging parents and her four dogs. Her husband worked a lot and she spent a lot of time alone. This is something she had grown used to over the course of their 29 years of marriage, but lately things had turned for the worse.

She knew there was something wrong when the things she used to enjoy in life weren't enjoyable anymore - like spending time with her animals and riding her motorcycle. She used to love caring for her dogs and the llamas but now they felt more like a chore than anything else, and she hadn't been on her motorcycle in over six months. She believed she was addicted to diet soda. That was what brought her in to see me. She'd drink up to 16 cans of diet soda a day. Chain drinking them like a smoker would light one cigarette with the end of another, she'd start opening a new can of soda before finishing the last drink of the other.

But it's OK she thought - because I'm a good caretaker, I take care of the home and animals, and it could be worse. I don't drink or anything like that. It's not that bad.

This is a dangerous line of thinking - "it could be worse", because what it does is allow us to settle - to not do anything and excuse our own feelings and desires away. And thankfully Cindy knew this was not the life she wanted. I have a lot of clients who employ this line of thinking, and I believe it's in part because we live in a world where people do have it worse - there's no argument there. And so clients don't want to seem as if they're ignorant to the true suffering in the world. I get that and appreciate it. But my belief is that each of us deserves to be truly happy, and excusing our happiness away because someone else has it worse is not the right approach. Think of it this way, if I'm feeling better, aren't I in a better position to help you? What about Cindy - if she's happier will she therefore be a better caretaker and spouse? Will she share her happiness with her friends and family just by being in a state of joy? Can she change the world merely by living her life to the greatest extent she can and modeling that behavior for everyone in her life? YES! I believe she can. We can teach our loved ones so many things just by being our best selves, not settling, and always striving for the best inside of us.

As the cans and cases of soda piled up, so eroded Cindy's self-respect and enjoyment in life. She gained 20 pounds in the course of two years and she was pretty sure the soda had a lot to do with it -because she found herself sitting down and drinking a soda instead of being active. And she had lost her spark, what mattered to her. She didn't feel like getting up in the morning and basically dragged herself through her work-day. She felt overwhelmed with all the work around her home that was piling up when she fell a little behind - not only did she need to take care of her four dogs, but she had the yard, llamas, and the home to take care of as well.

What was happening with Cindy was that she got in a funk and wasn't feeling good about anything. The diet soda wasn't helping her at all - it was merely a distractor. Thankfully, in hypnosis Cindy realized what she was really avoiding - problems in her relationship with her aging parents, and after realizing she needed to address her own insecurities with their failing health, she started feeling better. Her relationship with them didn't immediately turn around, but leaving it in a state of limbo and not accepting her new role in their life as a caregiver instead of their child was causing her so much stress she was drinking the soda to cope. But that just caused more stress because after gaining weight she didn't feel like being as active as she needed to be to care for them in the way they now needed her to -and that caused more stress in her relationship with them. She didn't like seeing them get older, but avoiding the situation wasn't helping at all.

Hypnosis helped Cindy realize what was really driving her behavior, and she was ready to make a change. The emotional work done in hypnosis gave her hope for a better future, but the issue of all that soda was still a problem. She had created an unhealthy habit. The soda was helping her not think about the stress with her parents- but it wasn't actually working.

The best way to stop thinking about something is to specifically think about something else - and the easiest way to do that is to do something else that required complete focus. If what we're doing requires all of our focus, there's no room for other thoughts to come in to play. This is one reason why many people like things that some would consider "dangerous" - like skiing, mountain biking, or in Cindy's case riding her motorcycle - because without complete focus on the task at hand there's a risk of injury or possibly death.

Cindy realized that although drinking the soda was temporarily taking her mind off the stress of her parent's health, it really wasn't working because the soda wasn't challenging enough to take her entire focus. So while she was sitting down drinking her soda, she was worrying about them and it was making things worse because she also tended to eat more and had gained that extra 20 pounds.

Instead, she committed to spending more time outside. She realized she wouldn't be able to ride her motorcycle as much as she wanted - it was a lot of work, and she had her actual paid job and other chores to do. So on days when she couldn't ride, she committed to spending time outside doing other things - just being in nature. Cindy realized that just by being outside she felt better. Some days she'd walk two miles, others she'd walk one and work in the yard for 30 minutes instead. Other days she'd spend a few hours riding after work. She added up how much time in her day was being spent drinking soda - almost two hours! And instead she spent it outside. She decided instead of binging on soda, *she'd binge on nature.* And it worked for her, and now even on days when she has time to only spend 10 minutes outside, she still does it. Because it's not always about the quantity of time she realized - it's just about consistently doing things that she loves to do. Now she can recharge herself with 10 minutes outside listening to the rain, or a short walk down the block and back. She tapped into her inherent power of renewal and recharge by spending time outside.

Now, Cindy has one soda per day with dinner. She drinks more water instead, and has lost almost all the weight she came in to lose. But it's so much more than that for her because she enjoys her days once again. Her parents' health issues aren't resolved, but they're better - because she's better. She spends more time with them, and feels better about helping them as they get older. She realized she had been stuck in a situation that wasn't going anywhere - she needed to change and face the reality of the situation. She is happier and more relaxed. She enjoys her days, which makes the energy in her home more relaxing and fun for everyone there. Hypnosis helped Cindy be happy being who she is right now by making a small change - a new default response by going outside and being in nature instead of drinking soda.

The next story is about a man named Terry who loved to distract himself from anger and back pain with potato chips. What you may find surprising and maybe even delightful is *the way* he creatively stopped eating the potato chips with the help of hypnosis.

Allergic to Potato Chips

Terry is a retired banker who was very angry. It was apparent in everything he said in our first session together. Angry at his brother and sister who were still alive and living in another part of the country, and angry at his mother and father who were both deceased. Issues over his father's estate amplified existing problems in the family that stemmed from years of growing up in an alcoholic household - eventually leading to Terry leaving at the age of 16 to live with his grandparents. But his father's ridicule and anger didn't stop because Terry left the house - the ridicule only transferred to his younger brother and sister.

Terry left his grandparents' home and joined the army as soon as he was old enough, but he unfortunately followed in his father's footsteps and struggled with anger and alcohol throughout his twenties. Thankfully, after his time in the service he met Shelia — his wife of 40 years.

Once he met Shelia everything changed, and he's had a good life for the last 40 years - but he's frustrated and worried because he still can't lose the last 15 pounds of weight he's been trying to lose for years.

Hypnosis helped Terry realize that old anger was still impacting his life. He realized this and noticed every time he was angry he'd reach for potato chips. Those potato chips took the edge off - even if it was only for a moment, but they were causing big issues in other areas of his life. With the power of hypnosis Terry was able to dissolve away the old, unactionable anger and he felt a lot better about himself and his life - but we also had to address the bad habit of eating potato chips when he was upset.

While in a state of hypnosis, I asked Terry what he'd like to do instead of eat chips the next time he felt upset. And to be clear, Terry was feeling much better about the long-standing unfairness and anger in his life, but the reality is that hypnosis is not magic and people still will experience feelings that we call bad - like anger and sadness. No matter how much hypnosis we do, life continues and stressful things still happen. So I knew in his future Terry would still feel angry or upset about something - and I wanted him to have a better response.

Note that asking this question while in hypnosis employs the deeper, creative, subconscious part of the brain that comes up with lateral solutions to the problems, solutions that we usually would not come up with otherwise. If I asked this same question outside of hypnosis, it would likely employ his conscious mind and the results would be limited - and usually these are the things clients come up with on their own anyway, and they haven't worked. Our conscious mind, being limited, does not always have the best answers to our problems.

In hypnosis, Terry realized that what really made sense to him was listening to music. He got out of the habit of listening to music because he just didn't enjoy it anymore. The newer technology was frustrating, and dealing with it just made him even angrier so he avoided the entire situation. But now that he was feeling better, he was willing to give it a try again.

Instead of reaching for the potato chips when he was upset, Terry agreed that his default response would be to put on some music - *even if he didn't "feel" like it at the time.* This is the trick with a default response - you have previously chosen it using your creative energy and wisdom, and agree to follow through without thinking about it. So whether you actually *feel* like doing it when the time comes or not doesn't matter - because you don't think about it. You just do it. So Terry just put on the music even when he didn't feel like it because he *knew* it was a better choice for him. Yes he is a smart man, and yes he had been accustomed to doing things in his life he didn't really *feel* like before too - like going to work every day in a suit and tie. He did it for other reasons. He was going to do this too. And listening to a song captivated him and took his mind other places, helping him to focus on other things. It didn't take but a few minutes for Terry to start feeling better. The interesting thing is that Terry often didn't realize that he was feeling better until much later - why? Because he was feeling better and was just enjoying listening to music. Later, he would recognize just how powerful choosing a default response was - so he started doing it for everything.

But Terry did something else that was so remarkable, and it really cemented this new habit in Terry's life - he applied a pattern that worked for him in other areas (being allergic to nuts) to eating potato chips. You see Terry was allergic to nuts - not deathly allergic thankfully, but if he ate nuts he would experience abdominal pain and cramping, so he avoided nuts completely. This was an easy choice for Terry - not one that he particularly liked because he did enjoy eating nuts (cashews specifically), but an easy choice to make given his body's response.

So he thought of potato chips in the same way -*as if he was allergic to them*. I asked him how potato chips made him feel, and his response was greasy and sluggish. They weren't contributing to his overall health and should be consumed in small quantities if at all. But it also led to other things. If he had chips in the morning he'd be more likely to continue eating other unhealthy foods the rest of the day. So in Terry's mind he realized that in a way, he was also allergic to potato chips - not in the traditional sense, but in a way that made him feel bad after eating them. In a way that helped him to choose not to eat them again.

Terry tried potato chips again before our last session, and admitted that he didn't really like them anymore - not like he used to. Since he had been eating healthier food the appeal wasn't there anymore and they really didn't taste as good to him. This happens because our taste buds change in about two weeks. This means with two weeks of healthier, cleaner eating, the junk food won't taste nearly as good - it may taste too fatty, or unnatural, too salty or sugary.

Over the course of our time together Terry lost almost 10 pounds, but the way he lost the weight was so interesting. A combination of getting rid of the anger, then selecting a new default response and thinking about chips as an allergen were unique and customized just for him. I didn't come up with these ideas - they were already inside of him.

Terry just tapped into a limitless powerful resource inside of him, and creatively applied the new elements into his life in a way that allowed him to easily change a bad habit to a good one. He took a pattern that worked for one area of his life, and applied it in a different way.

$\cdots\rightarrow$ PUTTING IT ALL TOGETHER $\leftarrow\cdots$

We think that in order to lose weight we have to work out at least 30 minutes a day, eat a healthy breakfast, three balanced meals, stop snacking, and basically eat perfectly. But it's just not true - not necessarily. Given the success stories with the many clients I've worked with, what matters most is finding a customized and creative solution that works just for you and your lifestyle and implementing it in a way to create a new healthy habit. And hypnosis helps us to find these customized solutions by bringing us self-awareness and insight. Perhaps a 30-minute workout daily is right for you - but maybe it's more realistic to walk or bike to work instead.

Understanding how habits work is an important aspect of learning how to change them, and the idea of a new default response is important because it helps us make it through that very important transitional phase of change. But if we really want to make healthy changes that last we have to learn to make daily improvements part of our routine - and that's what the next chapter is all about, how to make small changes every day with the power of Incremental Success.

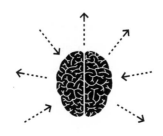

CHAPTER 5

Incremental Success

Be faithful in small things because it is in them that your strength lies.

- Mother Teresa

One of the biggest challenges with helping people lose weight is the fact that we still have to eat - it's not just the stopping of something to contend with, as in stopping smoking - although that certainly has its own issues, it's managing the food intake carefully. Too much and you can feel sluggish, tired and gain weight. Not enough, and you may feel a lack of energy and your body may put you in starvation mode and decrease your metabolism. And with losing weight the challenge can be much more complex in its implementation because we're managing something that our body needs to do every day in an environment that is heavily set up to keep us from being successful by surrounding us with unhealthy foods that are conveniently available. The healthier foods are often more expensive, take more work to obtain and prepare, and spoil more quickly.

Another challenge is the desire to want to see immediate changes - especially when we see commercials, testimonials, books and programs that promise huge and immediate weight reductions week after week. But those types of results are not realistic, nor are they sustainable. They may not even be healthy. The weight didn't come on in a matter of weeks, so it's unlikely to leave that quickly as well.

And that's why it's so important to realize a few very important aspects of losing weight.

1. Slow Weight Loss Leads to Permanent Results

First is that the faster you lose the weight, the more likely you are to gain it back. This is a common truth about weight loss, but the *why* is what really stands out as important to understand: if you are doing something drastic to lose the weight, then it is very likely not sustainable. If it's not sustainable you will either need to do something different to keep the weight off, or you will just gain it all back with old emotional, thinking, and behavioral patterns. This is why most weight loss experts recommend losing weight slowly - it's not necessarily because it's better for you, each person is different of course - it's just more realistic. If you learn techniques to consistently lose a little weight each and every day, you're much more likely to sustain that lifestyle and keep the weight off for life.

But let's just do a quick study on weight loss. I want to clarify how little we actually know about this, so the numbers are generalized. But it's believed that one pound = 3500 calories of food. So in order to lose one pound per week you'll need to have a 500 calorie deficit per day (3500 / 7 = 500). That deficit can come from either eating less food, or being more active or both. My recommendation is to be moderately active, and eat less. Mindful Eating, as discussed in chapter 1 will help your body to regulate how much food to eat. If you're really active, your appetite increases, and that can make it harder to lose the weight.

Back to the math, a 500 calorie per day deficit to lose one pound a week. If you want to lose two pounds a week that's 1000 calorie deficit per day, and so on. Five pounds a week is a 2500 calorie deficit per day, seven days a week. I hope you can understand how losing more than a few pounds a week really is NOT reasonable for the long term.

This is why when people go on crash diets, which are not sustainable, they easily gain all the weight back. The plans that enable you to lose weight quickly always involve some type of severe dietary deprivation so you feel as if you're starving yourself, or you're overexerting yourself with activity. Either way, it's not something most people can do permanently. And you don't have to.

A measured, sustainable approach is much better. But it can also be frustrating for clients because they have come to expect fast results that they've achieved with other programs or seen promised on television. And when I notice clients wanting rapid, unrealistic results I tell them they're welcome to do those other programs *again* and get *the same* results. Of course none of them want to. They want the permanent results, so they stick with hypnosis and lose a few pounds every week. But there's more going on than merely weight loss.

2. Focusing on the Entire Picture of Health Means Every Day Can Be Successful

Many clients come to me with their overall goal of losing the weight but when I ask them what is the benefit of the weight loss, they include elements such as:

✓ Sleeping better
✓ More peaceful: less worry, less anxiety
✓ More energy
✓ Increased self confidence
✓ Happier
✓ Better relationships
✓ Reduction in medication
✓ Increased mobility
✓ Less pain (knees / back / joints)

And so it's important to take into consideration ALL of the desired results throughout the whole process, not simply the weight loss. It's common just in the first few days of eating healthier for clients to sleep better and have more energy. So before the scale moves, there's already improvement and it's important to make note of those positive changes so you know you're moving in the right direction.

3. Focusing on Incremental Results Is a Powerful Approach for Continued Success

The best way to stay focused day after day, and excited and hopeful week after week is to focus on what I call incremental success. The hypnosis work often leads to huge insight and big leaps in awareness, improved emotional and mental processes and habitual change, *but it's the day after day improvements that keep clients going in the long run.*

One of the first questions I ask clients when I see them after the first session, which I learned from a good friend and hypnosis colleague Karen Hand, is "What worked for you this week?" This helps them focus on all the things they did right. The reality is that it's impossible to eat perfectly, and get exactly the right amount of activity every day - and we don't need to do either of those to lose weight. I've had clients that went from four candy bars a day to one and lost weight the first week. They went from eight beers a day to two and lost weight. And that type of change - incremental, is easier to implement and sustain.

One of the other questions I ask clients when the work is done is if they think they can continue like this - eating mindfully and getting moderate activity daily, plus the other customized changes we've come up with just for them - for the rest of their life? And they always answer yes. Then I'll ask if it's easier or harder than they thought, and the answer is always that it's easier - because they're not thinking about food as much anymore, not depriving themselves, and not working so hard.

And this point cannot be stressed enough. We want this to be as seamless and effortless as possible. The more you think about food, the more likely you are to eat. The more work it takes to measure, count, weigh, and plan the more you're thinking about food and the more likely you are to eat when you're not hungry. The more effort it takes you on a daily basis to eat healthy, the more likely you are to grow tired of the extra effort, and are much more likely to go back to old patterns if any stress comes up in your life.

Of course it's a balance. You need to do the planning in order to have healthy food available to you at all times - you need to shop for the healthy food -but after that, let your body tell you when it's time to eat. This is why it works so well for my clients. They get their life back and are spending time thinking about other things - sewing, gardening, working on their cars and projects; spending time with their grand kids and friends, and thinking less about food.

They get more life, less worry, move more, and eat less.

Incremental success is a powerful method for making any change we want to make in our life because when we focus on the small, daily changes that are feasible to make then the changes tend to be sustainable. Moments of insight that provide leaps in understanding are important as well, and insight is a natural part of good hypnosis work - but we can't count on those daily, so the foundation of continual change is incremental success.

These next stories highlight how hypnosis helped these clients find and then implement incremental success into their daily routine, which helped them to be successful with weight loss with minimal effort.

Jennifer Has Her Ice Cream and Eats It Too

Jennifer came to me because she had an ice-cream addiction - or so she thought. Every time she drove by the little store on her way home she felt compelled to stop in and buy a pint of her favorite vanilla bean ice cream and eat the entire thing. The problem was that it was such a habit that she had a hard time driving by the store without stopping, and she knew eating it regularly was not good for her - and by "regularly" she was eating nearly a pint a day.

Jennifer was still quite active, even though she was in her sixties. She had owned her own landscaping company and loved being outside working on one thing or the other, but had slowed down a bit as she'd gotten older.

Yet in her estimation she had gained over 10 pounds in the last six months, primarily because of this ice cream and she felt it had to stop.

She was still active, and ate relatively healthy. Her diet consisted primarily of whole foods - non-processed foods. I call these foods "food that your grandmother would recognize". Yet she was likely eating too much, in addition to the ice cream adding to her having too many calories in her day.

A week after our first session of hypnosis I asked Jennifer the question I always ask - "What worked this week?" I expect that much of what we cover in our first hypnosis session will work exactly as planned for my clients, and some things will need adjustment. This question helps clients to focus on what is working and the "not working" parts begin to fade away over time as there's an overwhelming amount of elements that work so well it crowds out everything else.

She told me that mindful eating was going really well. She had a harder time stopping when she was full, or satisfied, but it was almost automatic to eat only when she was hungry now. Instead of automatically having breakfast first thing, now she waited until her body told her it was time to eat - when she got a hunger signal from her body.

But she also said she "screwed up" with the ice cream. She stopped there once. "Just the once?" I asked, because previously it had been nearly daily. "Yes just the once, but the good news is that I didn't eat the whole pint. Actually I only had a few bites. It's still good, but it tasted overly sweet and rich."

She also noticed that she had lost weight, even in only one week her clothes were a little looser, and she had more energy during the day because she also wasn't eating such a large breakfast and she was sleeping better.

Overall she considered it a win. And in my estimation, a small serving of ice cream once a week IS the success I look for. That is incremental success. If we deprive ourselves of our favorite foods for too long, we're likely to binge on them. It's much better to be realistic and eat in a way that is sustainable. So I asked her if she could do that all over again, would she do it any different? Referring to the few bites of ice cream, and she responded that she wouldn't - because she had lost weight and it did seem easy to her. She didn't think about food as much, and yet she also wasn't depriving herself.

Her incremental success for that week was a reduction in overall food consumption, but more importantly from six pints of ice cream a week to 1/4 of a pint instead.

Yes, she still had her favorite ice cream, but now Jennifer also had the energy she wanted, the sleep she needed, and the peace of mind she was looking for. She now knows that as long as she just keeps doing what she did last week she'll lose all the weight she wants. And it's easier than she ever thought.

The next story is about a young woman who had a thriving social life and how insight gained during hypnosis helped her keep her friends, eat some tacos *and* lose weight at the same time.

Kelly Still Enjoys Happy Hour

Kelly came to me because she was worried she was drinking too much and was concerned for her future. She was single and had a high profile marketing job and a lot of friends - friends who liked to enjoy happy hour celebrations after work, and evenings spent eating and drinking.

But all the drinking and socializing was taking a toll on her. She loved running, and lately she wasn't enjoying it as much because she had gained 10 pounds and didn't feel like she had enough energy in the morning to run like she used to. She didn't drink enough daily to feel bad in the morning -and it wasn't impacting her job, so she didn't believe she had a drinking problem, but she didn't feel good about the way things were and she worried about her health in the future.

One of the issues that really stood out to her was her love of a Thursday evening Happy Hour tradition of Mexican food and margaritas. And lately her relationship with Thursday Happy Hour was feeling bittersweet because she was getting into a habit of having too many margaritas and tacos. She also noticed that when she drank, she was much more likely to over-eat.

Alcohol is not always a contributing factor when it comes to my clients who want to lose weight, but it is something I always ask about. Alcohol is certainly not a required substance - it doesn't provide us with anything nutritionally that we can't get elsewhere, so in many cases it's much better to abstain completely while on a plan to get healthier and leaner.

In Hypnosis Kelly discovered *why* she loved Thursday Happy Hour so much - it wasn't the food or margaritas she enjoyed, but the people - enjoying herself and spending time with her friends. The food was just an excuse to get together. Once she had that important insight, she was easily able to continue attending social events and focus on the intrinsic value of the activity - making connections, seeing friends, laughing, and enjoying herself. And the margaritas and tacos weren't necessary at all.

In the first week, Kelly didn't have anything to drink at all and she enjoyed herself so much - even more so in fact - that she decided to abstain from alcohol during *all* Thursday Happy Hours. She also eats smaller portions of the food and focuses on hanging out with her friends, laughing and enjoying herself. She didn't stop drinking entirely - she'll still have a glass of wine from time to time, but it's nowhere near where her drinking had been in the past.

One of the fears Kelly arrived with was - can I spend time with my friends that drink and still lose weight? And the answer is yes, not only for Kelly but also for many of my clients.

Some clients realize that many of their social events really aren't all that enjoyable without alcohol and they find themselves preferring to be outside walking or doing other activities either alone or with friends who are also wanting something different than the happy-hour bar scene. Many clients realize that they're not the only ones who want to be leading a more active and healthy lifestyle, so meeting for a walk or hike instead of a drink becomes more popular.

One of the best ways to keep up with your social calendar, but reduce drinking and eating unhealthy foods is to not draw attention to the changes. Most of my clients will order sparkling water with a lemon or lime, or they'll have water in a wine glass, then they just continue with their lives as normal. Drawing attention to the fact that you're not eating "that" (unhealthy) food or that you're not drinking for whatever reason will bring up insecurities or defenses in others around you and the consequences are likely not what you want. In Kelly's case, she still ate a taco on Thursday's Happy Hour, but didn't over eat. And she had sparkling water instead of margaritas.

She was surprised during the first Thursday where she made the switch that *no one even noticed*. They didn't ask why she wasn't drinking margaritas, nor about why she was eating less. Probably because they weren't really paying attention in the first place - not to that aspect of Kelly anyway. Most people are more concerned with their own behavior. If you don't make a big deal out of it, others may not as well. Or they may surprise you and ask why you're drinking and eating less and you can tell them because you have more energy when you drink and eat less, and that's what you prefer.

Now Kelly's life has changed - she is more active, but still has all the same friends. Two of them meet her now for walks regularly after work instead of happy hour. They're all happier for it. She still participates in Thursday Happy Hour, but now without the guilt, and also without the 10 pounds she had gained, because after two months she lost almost all of it.

Now she's happier because she has both her social life and the health and enjoyment she wanted. She didn't have to sacrifice one for the other, and she didn't have to give up tacos or margaritas entirely. She still enjoys them from time to time, and did when she visited San Francisco on vacation. She was especially happy that she didn't gain any weight on vacation either, as she usually had in the past. Her new way of living with incremental success, mindful eating and drinking, and keeping her social calendar and friends, with incremental modifications in her activity levels and caloric intake made the difference for her - and she already had the capability inside of her to make these changes.

I want to share Rob's story not only because it's inspirational, but also because it's very common. Many of my clients come to me after years of inactivity - yet with a history of being active, or athletic in younger years. What stopped them from being as active varies, but it's often a combination of: having kids, an injury or accident, a project at work that got out of control, or trauma - financial, physical or emotional. And the financial crisis in 2008 is what happened to Rob.

Rob Runs Off His Extra Weight in a 5k

Rob was an insurance broker and when the housing crisis of 2008 was in full swing he ended up losing not only his home but also his marriage. He moved across the country for a new job and to salvage what was left of his life, but in the meantime he wasn't active anymore and had put on over 20 pounds.

He missed his son and grandson, and wanted to visit them more often, but the last time he visited he could barely keep up with the 5-year-old, and it just made things worse because not only did he not live close enough anymore, but he believed he had let his physical body deteriorate while trying to keep his head above water financially. The insecurity of financial income loss, plus the lack of jobs in his local area left Rob feeling fearful for his future, and that was a feeling he was not accustomed to.

Hypnosis helped Rob first by removing erroneous fears about his past - the fear that he would go bankrupt which did not happen, and the fear that he'd be alone, which also did not happen. He wasn't with his wife anymore, but he realized in the end that ended up being a good thing and he was now dating someone new that he cared for very much. These unrealized fears can keep us trapped, and even if we don't realize they're there - the feeling of anxiousness or uncertainty can lead to behaviors such as inactivity, overeating and feelings of being out of control.

Hypnosis also helped Rob regain his self-confidence, and realize that some of the things in his life weren't really because of any one bad choice he made - likely anyone in his shoes would have made the same decisions. The decision that really bothered him was an investment he made that ended up turning sour because of the housing crisis, and that in turn caused him tremendous financial stress and arguments with his ex-wife which ended up leading to their divorce.

He's learned some things about himself and the decisions he made and feels more comfortable now. All of those elements were the underlying root emotional issue that would crop up when Rob wanted to run or ride his bike, which made him feel even worse, so once those feelings were dissolved through hypnosis, getting back into shape was easier because he felt better.

Rob wanted to jump back into his regular five miles a day immediately - but trying to start where he left off over a year and 20 pounds ago would likely be a mistake because it would be too much. One common mistake people make when trying to lose weight is they get excited and want to do it so quickly they start with something that really isn't feasible - like limiting themselves to a 500 calorie a day food intake and a two-hour workout. But that enthusiasm fades quickly, then they tend to give up after a few days and throw in the towel. The best approach is starting small and committing to something that is easily achievable each and every day, then slowly building up over time with incremental success.

Rob started with a 10-minute walk a day, but here's the trick. I asked him to commit to something that he could do even on his busiest day. So I asked him if even when he was really slammed at work, did he have 10 minutes? If not, then I'm not sure Rob would be able to prioritize himself in order to lose the weight to begin with, so this line of questioning is additionally beneficial because it gauges Rob's commitment to the change process and verifies he's ready to do what it takes.

He committed to 10 minutes a day, even on his busiest days. And just to be clear I have clients where I ask them to commit to one minute per day. Just. One. Minute. They can always do more. Here's why this technique works so well - they can get in the habit of doing this very quickly. No more "I don't want to run for an hour", or "it takes too long to get my gear together", or "it's cold and raining". Nope. You can do anything for one minute, and in Rob's case he could easily do it for 10. That's five minutes out the door, turn around and five minutes back.

The results I see with this style of incremental success are astounding. Clients stick to the one or 10 minutes a day, but usually end up doing a little more. But it's so much more than that because they *feel better about themselves, which leads to other incremental improvements in their life.*

Rob returned the next week, only one week later, and was up to two miles of walking a day. He wasn't running yet. When our time together was done, he was up to three miles a day of running and walking and had completed a 5k. He was getting back on track. He had also lost seven pounds and was feeling better than ever - more like himself he said. He scheduled a vacation to see his son and grandson again, and he had accepted an invitation to sit on a local board of advisors for a nationwide nonprofit organization that he cared about. Things had completely turned around for Rob, and it all started with incremental success backed with powerful hypnosis work to remove those limiting beliefs. Rob had it all inside of him, and with hypnosis he felt empowered to make the changes in his life he wanted to make.

···→ PUTTING IT ALL TOGETHER ←···

Incremental success is a powerful strategy for making any change you want to make in your life because it focuses on small, feasible improvements day after day. Here's an overview of how to get started in your life:

Step 1: Understand the Changes You Want to Make

The first step is to understand what changes you want to make and the best way to do that is to understand what the benefits are of the change you want to make? Do you want more energy? To lose 20 pounds? Reduce medication? Sleep Better? Fit into your favorite jeans?

Step 2: How will you know when you've improved?

The next step is understanding how you will *know* when it's improved? So many clients come to me and say things like they just want to be happier, or feel more peaceful, and when I ask them how they will *know* when they're feeling happier or peaceful they have no idea. Losing 20 pounds is easier to measure, but it's also very likely to take three or more months to accomplish, and we want to get you results now - so focusing on these other items is a great way to do that.

Take a moment to imagine, what would it be like if you were happier - what does that look like? Would you spend more time with friends? Take a vacation again? Write down a few characteristics of your increased happiness. What about when you're feeling more peaceful, what does that look like? Are you reading more? Riding your bike again?

Some people know they're feeling better when they're reading and interacting with friends and family. I'll give you a personal example: for me I know I'm happy when I'm reading a lot and listening to music.

Step 3: Let your Brain Do Some Work for You

Next, take a moment to imagine that you've already achieved these results. This is called starting with the end in mind, and there's a very good biological reason to do this.

Our brains have a system called the Reticular Activating System (RAS), which serves as a filter of the 400+ billion bits of information perceived by our senses at any one time.

Have you ever decided to make a big purchase, for example - a car, new computer, or home, then you begin seeing that car, computer or style of home wherever you go? That's RAS at work. What you've done is basically programmed your subconscious mind with the command that this new purchase is important to you, and the RAS elevates the priority of those elements to the top of the list - and does not filter them out, and you notice them more. The car, computer, home has always been there you just likely didn't notice it before because it wasn't important.

When you begin thinking about the benefits of the change you want to make, and what it looks like to get there, your RAS will begin filtering items in your environment that help you be successful. This is one of the very powerful ways that our minds help us make changes in our life, and when used properly - and especially with hypnosis, this type of programming can make the change seem easier than ever before.

For more information on reprogramming yourself for success including a downloadable template for implementing Incremental Success, check out the free online Reprogram Your Weight Toolkit that comes with this book at: ReprogramYourWeight.com/toolkit.

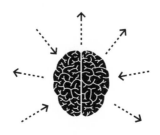

CHAPTER 6

Flow

May what I do flow from me like a river, no forcing and no holding back, the way it is with children.

- Rainer Maria Rilke

One of the secrets to being a great hypnotherapist is the following: even when my clients can't believe in themselves, I do. Even when they can't imagine being happy, or losing the weight, or being free from all the chaos and noise and frustration - I can. And I must. The moment I meet a new client I'm already creating for them in my mind and heart the future I can imagine where they're thinner, happier, and free. Where they're laughing and smiling, and noticing all the wonderful things already in their life they had somehow missed before. I can do that because I have years of experience proving to me that the hypnosis I do with them actually works - even when everything else has failed. And from that place, I gently guide each client into believing the same for themselves. Each and every week they move closer to themselves, discarding the emotional baggage that had been keeping them hostage for so many years, the limiting beliefs holding them back, and the habitual components keeping them trapped. Even through setbacks, they get closer to themselves. Once they're lighter emotionally, the physical weight begins to slip away and I get to meet the new version of my client - the one I've been waiting to meet all along. The one that walks into my office excited to tell me of all the changes she's experienced - both with food, but also with other aspects of her life too. And so what I've learned through this whole process is that hypnosis doesn't change people - not really, it helps them be rid of the things that were not theirs to begin with - it helps them return to themselves. I get to meet my clients, the real them, for the first time. And it's amazing.

How does that happen, you may be wondering? Well I believe it has to do with something commonly referred to as flow. Flow is a term used to describe an "optimal state of being". And I like to think of it as those moments in your life where time just slips away, and things are truly just flowing - effortlessly. There is an abundance and richness to your life - you may wake up in the morning and feel refreshed and energized, your coffee is more delicious than you remember, and everything you do unfolds with a joyful intent and impeccable timing. Everything around you seems brighter, more vibrant, and alive. You notice the butterfly as you walk by, and hear the birds singing. In a state of flow, you are in an optimal state of experience, and hypnosis can help you tap into this optimal state regularly, which is what you want because not only will you be feeling better and enjoying your life more than ever before but you will naturally eat less and move more which contributes to weight loss.

Getting into Flow

One of the reasons I love the concept of flow so much is that it can easily be described in emotional terms. Flow is a state of being where what you're trying to achieve is just outside of your comfort zone, but not so far that you feel overwhelmed. What this really means is that you can achieve a state of flow when what you're doing is a bit challenging - so you're not bored, but not so challenging that you feel frustrated and overwhelmed.

One of my favorite books on flow, *The Rise of Superman*, by Steven Kotler, references research indicating this optimal state is 4% out of our comfort zone. If what we're trying to do is 4% outside our comfort zone, we will likely be in a state of flow. If it's too far out, we will likely give up because it's overwhelming and frustrating. If it's too easy, we become bored and may reach for a bag of chips.

Here's how this applies to weight loss and getting healthier: just focus on getting 4% better each day. You will be in a state of flow. The changes in your life will feel effortless and they will become sustainable for the long term. Too many people want rapid change that puts them in the 25% range - it's too hard to only eat 500 calories a day for the long term. Too hard to work out for one or two hours a day, so what do they do? They give up. They chalk it up as another failed attempt at losing the weight. This is why I stress with my clients the importance of incremental success because that *is the 4%*. And when you can reach for that 4% day after day, you can begin living in a state of flow - living your life from one great moment to the next.

Flow is a state many clients achieve after their primary emotional hang-ups have been resolved - and this makes sense. They have to get rid of the initial problem first before they can move into that state of abundance that flow offers. This means I usually see hints of flow in my clients in the later part of our work together.

The following stories of clients are both inspirational, but also very unique in that these clients did not come to me asking for help getting into flow - they came to me asking for help losing weight and getting healthier. But what they learned along the way was something much more powerful, they learned how to tap into the best part of themselves and live in a state of optimal experience -regularly. Flow helps us lose weight because while we're in this state we're not emotionally eating. We're not feeling bad, or buying into limiting beliefs. We are in alignment with a greater part of ourselves and being fully present in the moment. This happens because hypnosis helps reveal to clients their inherent power within - and because it's within them, there's nothing else they need to do to have it.

Shirley Finally Jumps in a Puddle

Shirley had tried everything to lose the extra 30 pounds of weight she was carrying around, including all the popular weight-loss programs - but nothing worked for longer than a few weeks.

She came to see me because things were getting worse. Her husband had been diagnosed with a form of dementia, and she was feeling sad, lonely, and frustrated with the diagnosis. Her husband was slipping away from her each and every day. She missed her best friend, and it was hard when he repeated the same story or same comment to her over and over throughout the day.

She was also upset that the bulk of the work in their life was now up to her because her husband could no longer fix anything around the home like he used to, and he could not drive, nor do other chores such as pay the bills, or even cook. Even worse was that he didn't care to eat at home anymore, and preferred to eat out at restaurants every meal, a habit to which Shirley partially attributed to her weight gain.

But it wasn't just about Shirley, because her husband was gaining weight too. And when she was upset about something that he did or didn't do then she'd end up feeling guilty because consciously she knew he wasn't doing those things on purpose. He didn't forget where he put his glasses on purpose, he wasn't repeating himself on purpose. None of this was his choosing. And so she understood that she shouldn't be upset with him - yet she was upset, and it wasn't helping with the situation because there were fewer and fewer moments of happiness in their relationship and she feared the end of her life would be spent watching him slip away while she became more upset and frustrated.

Shirley's story is heartbreaking, and many of my clients come to me with similar stories that include deep suffering and pain. What they learn through hypnosis is that they're using food as a coping strategy - a soothing technique to feel better and take the edge off, yet it does not have the effect they want - it doesn't work. Instead they end up gaining weight, feeling sluggish and heavy, and it contributes to their current issues.

But what makes Shirley's story truly remarkable is the impact it had not only on her health and weight loss, but how it positively impacted every other area of her life as well. Many clients come to me to lose weight, but they often get so much more, and Shirley's story is a perfect example of that.

After the first session of hypnosis, I noticed a shift in Shirley's disposition. There was a smile on her face - a twinkle in her eye. She left the first hypnosis session a different person than when she came in.

The next week I saw her she reported some remarkable changes. She had started eating healthier when they ate out. This had some interesting consequences, because her husband naturally followed suit - she didn't order fries, and he didn't either. She ordered a salad and he did as well. She wasn't expecting him to start eating healthier with her - but he did. And in the first week she lost weight, and she believes her husband likely did as well, which was good for him since he already had limited mobility.

But it was so much more than that because week after week I witnessed Shirley truly coming alive. Shirley was experiencing moments of flow throughout her day where she was truly connected to the world around her - she was present in the moment - and it was helping her to lose weight because while in a state of flow she wasn't over eating. She wasn't even thinking about food, or her problems. Despite all the challenges in her life, she was overcoming them. Instead of being upset by the moments in the day where her husband was confused, she was noticing the moments of lucidity, laughter, and joy. She was focusing on the time they did have together, and because she was more joyful and happy, so was he.

The hypnosis helped Shirley tap into something that the other programs she had tried never did - it helped her to remember what *joy felt like* - and helped her realize that she could still experience happiness and joy - her life wasn't over yet. She was appreciating every moment of her day because hypnosis helped her to shift her perspective on life - she still had her husband, he was with her every day. She still had her health, her children, and happy memories.

Shirley started living her life from one joyful experience to another, and didn't really care about food anymore. As her focus shifted to more joyfully experiencing each day, her interaction with her husband improved. They were both eating less, and she was losing weight week after week. They still ate out often, but it was more for the company and enjoyment of being at the restaurant and interacting with other people than it was for the food.

On the last hypnosis session Shirley came to me and said "Erika, we're done. I don't need to see you anymore." Then she proceeded to tell me how much her life had changed from when she first met me. She told me a story to summarize her experience. When she was very young she remembers getting in trouble for jumping in a puddle: "proper young ladies don't jump in puddles" her mother had told her. And she realized how much of her life she spent thinking about what a "proper young lady" should do. She realized how much that held her back in her life. So last week, at the age of 71, she jumped in a puddle. Her husband looked at her astounded and asked, "what are you doing?" "I'm enjoying my life," she replied. And she dried off her shoes, but kept on her pants covered in specks of mud the rest of the day, because a "proper older woman" would never do that. And she's done being proper.

"Erika", she continued, "in that first session something shifted for me and I didn't really know what it was at the time, but now I do…I know what it is now. I remembered what it felt like to *feel alive*, to laugh, to sing, to dance, to look forward to things - to be excited. And so that's now where I'm living my life. And each day there is something to look forward to, and I get better as I learn to live with my husband and his diagnosis but I've learned that laughter is such a powerful medicine. That is true, so we laugh every day. We jump in puddles, look for rainbows, and enjoy each other as much as possible."

Shirley was living her life in a state of abundance and flow - noticing all the good around her. As she did that, the problems seemed to dissipate, and she naturally ate less as her focus was on the entire world around her.

The next story is about Kim, a woman who suffered a terrible loss but was able to find the strength within to move through her grief and begin to enjoy her life again. With hypnosis she not only found the insight to heal quickly, but she also tapped into her true power of resiliency - moving way beyond weight loss to creating a life she wanted.

Kim Starts Singing Again

Kim was almost 150 pounds overweight when I met her, and she was sad. That's the only way I can describe how Kim was feeling. Deep sadness and longing for someone she lost long ago - her first and only child.

Kim and her husband lost their little girl to an illness when she was only two years old, and this had caused years of suffering and struggle within her emotionally, but also in her relationship with her husband. She waited to try to have another baby because the suffering was so great, and now she believed it was too late. She knew she was an emotional eater, and that her grief surrounding the loss of her baby was driving her to eat for the wrong reasons and gain weight. However, knowing these things was not enough, regardless of what Kim understood about her problem she couldn't figure out anything that would actually help her to feel better. She had tried everything she could think of with limited results.

Hypnosis first helped Kim by helping her come to terms with her situation. She had been trying for so long to fix her problem by just not thinking about the grief. By staying so busy doing other things, there really was no space in her head for being sad. But that technique was not working, and it was apparent the moment I met her and she burst into tears. The sadness was just barely under the surface, Kim was putting on a front of being happy and joyful, but that's not how she really felt inside. Behind the smile on her face was deep sorrow that had yet to be addressed.

Kim was courageous enough to face her grief and loss, and hypnosis helped Kim move through that painful experience very quickly. I learn a lot from my clients, they teach me things every day. And Kim is an example of a client who through her own creative abilities was able to find a way to help herself move beyond the grief and find something else to love, another dream to accomplish.

I first noticed Kim in a state of flow at the end of her third hypnosis session when she sang a song- not a very long one, just a few phrases. But it was a song that came from deep within. And it was about her own faith that there is a plan for her life and her future. But the song itself was astoundingly beautiful and I could tell she was in a flow state as she sang it. Have you ever experienced someone so overcome with positive emotion just begin singing? That is what happened to Kim. Then she told me how she used to sing - all the time, but the singing hadn't felt right to her for a very long time. Her heart wasn't in it. But now is the time, she told me, to start singing again.

When Kim sang, it helped her to express herself and live her life more joyfully. It helped her to feel feelings of sadness and pain, and move through them. It helped her break her habit of using food to numb her feelings and live her life to the fullest. Kim started singing again with her group, but her singing spread out to all other areas of her life as well. She allowed herself to feel things more deeply again. When we try to keep ourselves from feeling things like grief and sadness, we block out the good emotions as well, including joy and happiness. And Kim's avoidance of feeling her grief was holding her back from feeling joy and happiness.

Kim continues to lose weight week after week, and she knows it will take time to lose all 150 pounds, but she knows it's going to happen now. And she looks for ways to make her life better every day, just a little bit. Then she sings about them.

The next story is about John. Through hypnosis John was able to lose weight and spend more time doing the things he loved - which included being with his grandson. There's an interesting twist to John's story that demonstrates the true power we all have for resiliency - and maybe even grace.

John's Story: Seeing Things Differently

John had a hard life, there was no denying that. At 63 his body was broken in places from years working for the local transportation company. It was difficult, laborious work, but he enjoyed it. But now he had a back issue from an injury, and in the past he had struggled with prescription medication to help ease the pain. He traded in his addiction of pain medication for a sugar addiction, and now was over 40 pounds overweight, which only increased the pain in his back and reduced his mobility and quality of life even further.

John was thankful he was no longer addicted to pain medication, but it was not easy for him to get through his day. The only time he actually enjoyed himself was when he was eating.

This is the sad but honest truth about many of my clients - the moments when they are eating are the most joyful of their days. While eating they are happier, and without worry. Yet a common belief is that overweight people are lazy or without will power, and that's not my experience at all. The people I help lose weight are smart, thoughtful, creative and kind. They've just often been dealt a bad hand so to speak.

But John's story isn't just about his physical pain, it's also about his relationship with his own father who was an alcoholic and belittled him every chance he got. John grew up in a household where he was made to feel no-good, worthless, and literally told by his father nearly every day of his young life that he wished he had never been born.

John was determined to make sure his own kids never felt the same way, the way he did, so he showered them with love and affection. And it worked really well. His kids felt loved and appreciated, and John was happy that he was able to do for his own kids what his father never did for him.

The problem was that now John was a grandfather, and it was difficult for him to spend time with his grandson because of his back pain, so instead they'd go for donuts and ice cream. This is where John really got into trouble because he built a very bad habit of eating donuts every morning - with his grandson or not, and ice cream or dessert every evening.

John had tried everything to lose the weight, but because he couldn't move very much, he naturally wasn't very active. And he had a habit of eating a lot of food. After years of hard work, he was used to eating a big breakfast, a big lunch, and a big dinner. Yet with his physical limitations, his body didn't need that many calories anymore.

Hypnosis first helped John tap into the power he *did have* inside of him - things that he had not been aware of before. It helped him to overlook his physical limitations, and find other things he *could* do that brought him joy and wouldn't cause him to gain weight at the same time. This was a shift in thinking for John that in later sessions would lead to a state of flow because it helped him to be more active and enjoy his life more - even if the activity was different than what he had been used to.

And what is remarkable about John's story is that once he was able to let go of the anger and frustration at his father, his perception of pain dissipated as well. He realized he was using his pain as a point of focus to remain angry with his father for years of abuse - because both things were unfair. The way his father treated him was unfair, as was the injury that led to his back pain. And they were linked in his mind. Once he realized being angry with his father was only hurting him, he chose to let it go and not be angry. Letting go of anger is often easier in a state of hypnosis because clients can actually feel the anger and notice the associated beliefs that go along with it. Then we use techniques to help them release that feeling and gain insight into what the anger was intending to address, and then they can equally feel when the anger is gone. In John's case, he understood that his father was an alcoholic and was suffering in his own way. He knew this now at an even deeper level because of his own struggles with prescription pain medication. And with that realization - knowing it really wasn't about himself at all but about his father's own limitations and struggles - John felt better. His back didn't seem to hurt as much.

John knew his life would never be the same as it had been before his back injury, but he also knew he had a lot going for him. He started eating healthier and listening to his body when it came to his appetite and hunger. And he started losing weight right away, but that didn't mean it was easy. It did take some getting used to, and one thing that helped was while he was in hypnosis, John realized something very important that hadn't been apparent to him before - all the other things in his life he could do, including things with his grandson.

Through hypnosis John was first able to move beyond anger, then beyond pain, and from there he was able to enter a state of flow, which for him was all about appreciating everything around him he already had. Now John looks at life from a place of abundance - an abundance of love for his kids and grandkids. Not from a place of scarcity or lacking anything. He no longer wakes up in the morning dreading the day and wishing for times before he was injured - instead he looks forward to each day. John started doing more each and every day, looking for his 4%. "How can I get better today?" he told me he asks himself every morning.

He discovered photography and drawing. He took his grandson on short walks and they took pictures and learned to draw the world around them. This was much more satisfying than eating donuts and ice cream, because they had meaningful discussions about life and what they saw in the natural world.

Hypnosis helped John actually *look* for ways to make his life better - to see it through art and photography. To live life to the fullest, even if he could only walk short distances. And now he does look for the 4% every day, wondering how he can capture the bluebird out his window more artfully, or what about the picture of the sunrise, could he do a better job of crafting that image?

John still enjoys an occasional donut or ice cream, but neither really mean the same to him anymore. Now he's looking for new things in his life to enrich his experience, and he's happier and more peaceful than he's ever been.

John is half way to his weight loss goal, but it's so much more than that because he has a new perspective on life. Even when his back hurts, it doesn't bother him nearly as much, and he has new techniques to help him enjoy his life without causing him to gain weight.

Each of us may have physical, financial, or other challenges, but when we focus on what we can do, we'll make improvements. Hypnosis helps us see life from that new, updated perspective.

Where's My 4% Today?

One of the most important things I learn from my clients is how to be resilient, how to find the silver lining - the underlying positive lesson in life's experiences - and how anything that we love and find joy in can help us be successful.

Look for ways to improve your life - just a little, look for that 4%. Don't overdo it, over committing often leads to frustration and ultimately failure. Set yourself up for success and find something just outside your comfort zone, but not so far that you feel overwhelmed. Allow yourself to find creative solutions to issues in your life; they are often the ones that will truly help shift your experience in the direction you want your life to go. No cookie-cutter solutions here. The best ones are ones made especially for you. And how do you come up with them? By reaching deep down inside and tapping into your own power within - your own inherent power.

Achieving a state of flow helps us lose weight and so does the topic of the next chapter: seeing food for what it really is.

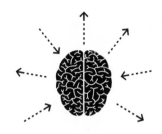

CHAPTER 7

See Food for What
It Really Is

Absorb what is useful, Discard what is not, Add what is uniquely your own.

- Bruce Lee

For many of my clients, what they come to realize is that in their life they have elevated the importance and role of food to such a high degree, that it really is being used in ways food is not designed for. In their minds, food is placed on a pedestal as the fixer of all things - Feeling sad? Eat ice cream. Lonely? Popcorn and a movie. Upset? Happy hour appetizers and drinks. Not sure what that bad feeling is? Definitely a drive-through type of night.

Food is not meant to fix all of our problems. It's primarily meant to bring our bodies nourishment and energy, and of course some pleasure. Yet, many of us are taught when we're young that a scraped knee can be fixed with a cookie, or at a young age that an ice cream sundae can help us when our bunny passes away. And it can help, a little, but food is not designed to fill an emotional hole.

Meeting for dinner or drinks is a common social activity, but often the underlying intention is to spend time with loved ones. But sometimes we focus more on the food, and less on connecting with others.

These types of scenarios regarding food are everywhere. And there's really nothing wrong with these scenarios either - until it turns out that they're negatively impacting our life. Then it's important to look at food and our relationship to it with an updated perspective.

The reality is that for some of these minor issues - like a scraped knee, food can help us feel better. It can take our minds off the minor sensation of pain, as long as it wasn't that bad to begin with, until it subsides. The danger lies in taking that solution and trying to apply it to other, bigger issues in our life - such as turning to food to fill a longing for human acceptance or connection, for example. Trying to use food to solve a big problem like loneliness just causes stress and frustration because it does not work - food can't fill an emotional need like that. You may feel better for a moment, but in the end, you'll be left feeling overweight, frustrated, and out of control.

Hypnosis helps to put food back into its proper place by helping us see it for what it really is- energy and nutrition for the body. It can also be pleasurable - but it shouldn't be our only or primary source of pleasure. It's possible to still enjoy food and lose weight at the same time - it's a balance. Many societies and traditions use food for celebration and social interaction, and again there's nothing wrong with that—unless you have an issue with food. Just as there's nothing wrong with having a beer unless you have a drinking problem. If you do have a problem with food, then expecting it to do anything more than meet the needs of your physical body is just going to cause you ongoing problems and frustration.

The following stories demonstrate how hypnosis enabled these clients to see food in an updated, healthier way.

Saying No to Emotional Eating Is a Yes to Everything Else

Joel worked for the state as an accountant and he travelled regularly as a part of his job. On any given day Joel could drive 10 minutes or 200 miles to various work locations. It was hard for him to eat healthy on the road with such a diverse and challenging schedule, and it had caused him to gain 15 pounds over the last year.

Joel was also an avid cyclist and led a local cycling group on weekend rides. But he was becoming increasingly embarrassed as a team leader because of his weight gain, and it was also slowing him down.

He was feeling frustrated because in the past, if he gained a few pounds all he would need to do was be a little more conscience about his eating, ride a little more, skip the beer after work, and he'd lose the excess weight. But this time even that wasn't working, because he didn't feel like riding anymore - it was too much work to drag his cycling gear around to all the various locations he travelled to, and he was tired at the end of the day. He found himself more often than not just going back to the hotel room with some fast food or visiting a local bar for dinner and a beer.

Joel's experience is very common - so many of my clients are working so hard in one way or the other that they don't have the energy left to make the healthier choice. It takes time and energy to eat healthy, whether you're at home or on the road. And it takes time and energy to be active - and both of those are more challenging if you're working hard in other areas of your life.

Hypnosis brings us clarity about issues in our life that we may have overlooked in the past - things that deep down we may know, but haven't risen up to our conscious awareness. Through hypnosis Joel realized that he was in the habit of eating unhealthy food when he was on the road. This had been going on ever since he could remember. Since he was a young boy, whenever he travelled with his family they always ate out at restaurants, and he got to eat the "bad" food they weren't allowed to eat at home - he ate dessert and candy nearly every night, and had French fries almost every day. Yet now as an adult he realized he was doing the same thing - eating poorly while on the road. It was a reward for working hard in the day, a treat - just like when he was younger. But he also realized he had a choice. He realized that there were many things in his life that he did when he was younger but didn't do any more - like sleep in a bunk bed, or believe in the Easter bunny. Many of the items he did when he was younger just didn't work for him anymore - and this was just one of those things.

Joel decided that instead of saying 'Yes' to the unhealthy eating habits when he was travelling and giving in to his desire to reward himself, he was going to say 'No' instead. No to the junk food. No to the fries. No to the beer and eating out because in saying No to those things, he gets to say Yes to every other thing in his life that actually mattered to him - to losing the weight, to feeling good about himself, to getting excited and looking forward to cycling again, to appreciating his role as a team leader.

Through hypnosis, Joel also obtained a more realistic perspective on his relationship with food. He realized that he was the only one putting food in his mouth. The choice was his, and because it was his choice, he also had all the control. Although he enjoyed eating that type of food when on road trips as a kid, it wasn't right for him anymore. He'll always treasure those old memories with his family eating fun foods, but now he's making a different choice - a grown-up choice that fits his lifestyle. Once Joel started seeing unhealthy junk food for what it really was, and what it was doing to his life, he wasn't interested in it anymore- it actually didn't even appeal to him.

The best part for Joel is that he had everything inside of him already to do this - he just started seeing food in a new way, a more realistic and healthy way that enabled him to easily eat healthier on the road and get everything else in his life he wanted at the same time.

The next story is about Tina and how she was able to reprogram herself with hypnosis to stop thinking about food so much, which helped her start losing weight right away - while also giving her peace of mind and changing her relationship with food.

Food and Eating Take a Backseat to Life

Tina worked for a local computer company and sat in her cubicle on the phone and computer nearly all day long. She had what she considered a good marriage and a good job, but there was something missing from her life.

She came to see me because she felt out of control. Every moment of the day she thought about food - she would go from eating one thing to the next while sitting at her desk. From yogurt, to pretzels, to an apple, then lunch. After lunch she'd have a protein bar or some nuts, then check out the break room to see if there was anything new there to eat. On her way home from work she'd stop and get a large diet soda or iced tea and maybe some fries, or take-out, then have dinner and continue eating the rest of the night as she watched television. She was desperately out of control and felt that food was taking over her life.

Part of working in a cubicle environment is the lack of privacy and ease with which everyone can hear everyone else's conversations. And the conversations were not helping Tina with her goal of losing 80 pounds - her colleagues were constantly talking about food - what they had for dinner, what they're having for lunch, where they're going to eat over the weekend, and what unhealthy food was waiting to be discovered in the break room.

All of this talking about food was causing her to think about food all day long. For Tina, it was to the point where not only her time at work, but also her entire life revolved around what she was eating next- where were her and her husband dining that evening? What was for lunch tomorrow? Where should she get dessert for this Sunday's dinner with her parents?

So many of my clients have similar issues with food - over time food slowly becomes the center of their existence, yet they don't always realize it. Actually at times it seems normal. Food *is* everywhere, and it's a common go-to activity for social events as well. And food is easy - after a long day at work, many people don't want to do anything other than relax or eat. Going on a hike, or working on a project just doesn't sound good anymore at the end of the day. So often plans in the evening are all about what's for dinner. Weekends can be much of the same - checking out the new restaurant, plans with friends or family at a local pub, baking cookies or a cake for a party. For many of my clients it's almost as if their hobby or extra-curricular activity is food in one way or another.

Hypnosis works in these cases by bringing a much-needed reality check to daily living. And for Tina, hypnosis provided her clarity and a new perspective. She could now understand that in her life food was playing much too large of a role - it was not only feeding her, but it was also keeping her from being bored at work, and it was her nightly and weekend entertainment. She wasn't able to recognize this before because she was just living her life, and the changes occurred slowly over time. Now she recognized that her reliance on food as an activity had actually pushed out all the other things in her life she used to enjoy doing - like antique shopping with her husband, needlepoint and crossword puzzles at home, and making quilts for a local charity. Food had replaced all of those activities- she just had the one thing she was doing - and it all revolved around food and eating.

After this shift in Tina's perspective, food took on a new role. She told me she started "tuning out" her co-workers' discussions about food. Interestingly, she didn't do this on purpose, meaning she didn't actively try to tune them out -Tina's subconscious naturally started tuning out discussions of food. Instead of following along with her co-workers ongoing discussions of food related items, Tina's subconscious was tuning into a new station for her - pointing her in the direction that she wanted to go. She was daydreaming about the walk she was going to take after work. She started doing crossword puzzles on her break instead of checking out the food in the break room. Her subconscious mind was highlighting activities and events she would be interested in that had nothing to do with food.

Tina started losing weight right away, but she was more surprised by how easy it was for her mind to shift to thinking about other things. This shift - tuning into her new station, made the change easy for her, which helped her be successful right away and stick with being healthy and active over time.

Shifting our perspective at the subconscious level is one of the powerful aspects of hypnosis, because when we make changes at that deep level we can actually see and hear things differently - what's filtered and brought to our conscious awareness changes. This means we've altered the perception of our reality in real-time by filtering out what we don't want. No longer do we notice the donuts in the break room -we may not see them at all. It doesn't mean they're not there - we just don't notice them. No longer do we pay attention to the billboards advertising a fast food restaurant, or the commercials - they don't make it past our new subconscious filter. Hypnosis can help us see food for what it really is in our life, then put it where it should be - there for energy and nutrition and sometimes pleasure as well. Then it helps us to notice the things that help us achieve that goal. This is how with the aid of hypnosis weight loss can seem easy - because you employ the use of your subconscious mind to filter out everything that is not helping you.

But we can't filter out food entirely from our awareness. We do in fact need to think about food to some extent in order to be successful in losing weight, and that's the focus of this next story: balancing our thinking and planning of food for consistent healthy eating.

A Little Planning Goes a Long Way

The previous stories highlighted different ways clients realized food was taking on much too large of a role in their life and how they put food back into a healthier, more realistic place. But what does that really look like? How can we balance food in our busy lives in an ongoing way that helps us both eat healthy, but not focus on it so much that it becomes all-consuming?

The answer is planning and balance. I want you to think about anything big that you've accomplished in your life that has been successful. Perhaps graduating from college, or completing a challenging work project, buying a home, or even throwing a large party like a wedding. Most of them involved some sort of planning. Yes, it's possible to throw an ad-hoc party, or to "be in the right place at the right time" type of situation when buying a home, but even those scenarios are often supported by some level of pre-planning -already having some savings ready for a down payment, for example.

The point is that for many of the really important things in our life we do a fair amount of planning, and successful weight loss is the same way. The challenge is that if you are doing too much planning, you end up thinking about food all day long, which can increase your appetite and cause you to gain weight. And too much planning can begin to feel like a part-time job, which is not what we want since the effort to maintain that is not sustainable.

Instead, a better approach is a focused amount of planning and preparation, then nothing more. Hypnosis offers a huge advantage when it comes to planning and preparation because while in a state of hypnosis, clients imagine their future - they program their subconscious mind with the future they want. They imagine doing the activities that lead to weight loss, like grocery shopping for healthy food and eating healthy meals, and they also imagine themselves as having already lost the weight. They see themselves a smaller size and imagine walking around in their lighter body.

Hypnosis offers clients the ability to program the subconscious mind and say, "here, this is the path we're on, this is where we're headed". And just like the story of Tina reprogramming her mind to tune out her co-workers, clients can reprogram their subconscious minds to focus on being active, happy, and eating healthier. Then follow-through when the time comes is much easier, because hypnosis helps set an expectation for success.

One of the mistakes I see clients make over and over, is thinking about what they don't want instead of thinking about what they DO want. And this is an important aspect of any change we want to make in our lives. Only think about what it is you do want to take place. Whether you're in a state of hypnosis or merely daydreaming or thinking about what you're going to do later, only think about what you DO want to happen. The mind does not think in negatives, this is why if I said to you don't think of a purple hippopotamus, you first need to think of it before you cannot think of it. So imagine yourself as if you've already achieved your goal, and you'll be more successful. If you say to a child, for example "don't spill the milk" over and over they're much more likely to spill the milk. A better approach is to say, "be careful with your milk", because it's what you actually want them to do.

At a minimum, I recommend that clients plan to have healthy foods available to them at all times - this means in their home, at work, and when on the go. Then they wait for a hunger signal from their body to eat. The body is the best indicator of when to eat. I also recommend that clients plan on being active every day. A good rule of thumb is to know the day before what activity you will be doing the following day. Don't leave it up to the day-of as it likely won't get done because other activities will get in the way.

Plan to have healthy food available, eat mindfully, and know when you're going to be active, but also know that plans change. And that's fine - it's expected that plans will change. Think of your plans as heavily penciled in - by that I mean not easily erased, but possible to erase and change. And that's what Cheryl discovered in her weight loss journey - a change of plans can be a good thing.

Cheryl was about to retire from a business she had created and owned for over 30 years. Technically she was selling her practice to someone else, and she was looking forward to her future life spent gardening, travelling, and spending time with her friends.

But she was concerned about her weight, and knew that a decrease in her activity and more free time on her hands when she retired meant she might gain more.

Cheryl was definitely a planner - she had planned out her retirement and the sale of her practice for years. She planned her vacations months in advance. But she didn't plan on staying healthy and thin - and because of that lack of planning she ended up gaining weight. She told me she ate "whatever" for breakfast and had lunch at her desk most days. She didn't plan her meals, nor have much of anything healthy to eat at home. This had actually worked for her for quite some time until she was in her mid-forties, then she started gaining weight.

Cheryl had tried other things to lose the weight, but none of them worked for very long because of her hectic schedule. She didn't have time to put into careful management what she was eating on a daily basis. So hypnosis helped Cheryl create a realistic plan for her healthy future. She was able to "try on" different scenarios while in hypnosis to understand if they would actually work for her. While in a state of hypnosis she could access all the underlying emotional and mental components that went along with her daily activity. She realized that coming home from work to cook dinner would not work for her. That could not be a part of her plan. She could, however, make crock-pot meals or enchiladas on the weekend and eat those throughout the week. She could also have fruits and vegetables already cut and in her fridge for an easy salad after work or to put in a bag for lunch. Hypnosis helped Cheryl first see the food for what it really was - a necessary component of everyday living. Just because she wasn't planning for it didn't mean the food wasn't there. She had to eat, and by not planning, she ended up making choices that weren't healthy for her. So instead Cheryl made minimal plans for shifts in her life that could contribute to her success.

The amazing thing about Cheryl's story is how easily she implemented her new plan into her life. No, things didn't go perfectly - some days she didn't feel like eating the stew or enchiladas and still picked up something on the way home. But what she picked up was healthier than before - more in line with her new way of thinking and new way of eating. She found that just a little bit of planning and preparation all week helped her not only eat healthier more consistently, but she also realized how much time and energy she *had been* putting into eating. In the past when she was hungry and didn't have anything, she'd have to leave the office and go downtown to get some food or to the grocery store. Now that she had food with her, not only did she eat healthier, but also the food actually saved her time. She realized that on some level, she didn't plan her meals because she wanted and needed that break from work - she wanted to leave and go get the food. It was a good excuse that she could accept. But once she started planning better, she realized she could not only eat healthier, but that she really did need to take a break and she didn't have to leave the office to do that.

Now Cheryl is putting less time and effort into eating, she's more effective at work, and she's lost over 30 pounds in about six months.

She planned to lose the weight, and it worked. Cheryl started seeing food for what it really was - not an afterthought, but something that is necessary in life and something she could plan for in order to be healthy, lose weight, and have the energy she desired to do other things.

⋯→ PUTTING IT ALL TOGETHER ←⋯

Food plays an important role in our lives - to nourish and energize our bodies, as a source of pleasure, and as a point of focus for social gatherings and entertainment. But many people use food in other ways that it's not designed for and that causes unwanted consequences, like using food to soothe us emotionally. And although food works in the short run to alleviate unwanted feelings, the changes are always temporary - the hurt feeling returns and we likely gain weight in the process.

Seeing food for what it really is helps us to reset the role it's playing so we can eat healthier and feel energized, sleep better, and feel good about ourselves. When we eat the right way for our body, we feel vibrant and full of vitality. In the process of paying closer attention to our relationship with food, we'll often notice places where we're eating and it's not having the desired result, and in that case we're given information that we can use to make better choices to get the results we want. Either way - we win. We lose weight and have more energy while we find new ways to experience pleasure and enjoy social gatherings. We change our relationship with food in a way that helps us eat healthy, lose weight, and feel good for the rest of our lives.

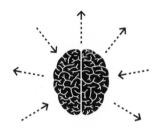

CHAPTER 8

Tapping into Your Inherent Power with Hypnosis

You are not a drop in the ocean. You are the entire ocean in a drop.

- Rumi

I wrote this book because I see so many of my clients struggle with their weight and I want to help as many people as possible with a message of hope. The message is that each of us has the power already inside of us to lose weight and keep it off for good. If you've tried everything with limited results, does it make sense that there may be something deeper going on? I think so. And if you've "thought" about this issue as much as you can consciously, and still aren't getting the results you want, then know that hypnosis will give you even more information - at the subconscious level. But hypnosis won't just give you more information, it will also shift how you feel about things. And when we *feel* like eating healthier, and being more active it's much easier to follow through. Actually, it can begin to feel effortless.

What is the relationship between inherent power and hypnosis you may be wondering? Our inherent power is always there. We have all this information inside of us from our life's experiences. Some people call it intuition or a gut reaction, but many times that information is coming from the subconscious mind. Hypnosis brings us clarity and that's why it works so well -with more information and a new understanding we know *how* to make any change we want to make. We understand *why* it wasn't working in the past.

The power is in the information that is within us - in our subconscious mind - we just have to figure out a way to tap into it. We can do that naturally in moments of insight during our everyday lives - sometimes during a hike, a drive, or while working on the yard, or in times of crisis or tragedy. I like hypnosis because we can capture that knowing in the subconscious mind without having to do any of that, and hypnosis is repeatable. When a client walks through my door I *know* I have the techniques to help them.

Hypnosis helps us in these two ways.

- It enlightens us to the reality of our situation. This new information and insight resolves the emotional underpinnings that we often didn't realize were there. We feel better, we feel lighter, and we have clarity.

- We use hypnosis to imagine the future we want. We program that in with powerful hypnotic suggestion, and with that expectation of success, we are able to follow through on things and do things as we want.

Hypnosis is not magic. And your hypnotist does not have all the answers - *but you do*. Whether you realize it or not your solution is within you. Why is that? Because you are an individual, a unique person. And some of the solution for you will be understanding what's holding you back, and some of the solution is understanding how to move forward. That's the job of a hypnotist - to guide you to your own solution, a unique and custom solution that will work just for you and your lifestyle. And a good hypnotist knows the tools to get you into a deep state of hypnosis quickly, then tools to uncover what's holding you back, and others still to help reprogram you to move forward. A good hypnotist can help bring you that clarity, and point you in the direction you want to go.

I know you can do this. I've seen hundreds of clients walk through my door sad, depressed, and nearly broken. They're done. They say, "Erika, I don't know why I'm here, I've tried everything else. I'm tired. I hope you can help me". And they are surprised by the results. Because we always discover something about them that they didn't realize was happening - something that perhaps happened long ago that they "thought" was resolved but wasn't. Or a limiting belief or feeling that was keeping them from being successful. Or just a way of thinking that was stunting progress.

My goal is for you to be successful. To be happy. To find the peace and joy and happiness in your life. To feel good about your body, to feel a lightness in your step, to reconnect with joyful activities, people and events on a daily basis. When you do that you can share it with the world and be an even better partner, parent, sibling, colleague, business owner, citizen - a better human. We can all make the world a better place, first by starting within. By discovering what's going on inside, connecting with our inherent power, then sharing our unique gifts with the world.

ACKNOWLEDGEMENTS

When I was young I had dreams where I would build a plastic plane, and fly above my home in it. Sometimes I would take the plane really high and fly into the blackness where it was quiet, and the stars lived. I would swoop and twirl in my plane.

The feeling I had in these dreams was amazing - a feeling of limitless freedom and joy.

Later on, without realizing it, I met people who gave me that same feeling. They were my teachers in life, and they believed in me and supported me and made me feel like I could do anything.

First were my parents. My father who taught me to play games – games of my own creation. He's the man that created the "Froggy Book" with all our collective ideas. We'd open the Froggy Book and pick a game we had created to play. Later he taught me to love the freedom of a convertible, and that you don't really need to have a destination in a car with the top down. A sunny day, and wind in your face is enough.

My mom taught me to create in another way – she modeled kindness and compassion. She loved through not only words, but also action. She helped me bake a cake for a new student who felt left out. She understood why it was important to me that everyone felt loved – because she's the one that taught that to me.

Later in life I had teachers that gave me a quantum leap in my own personal growth – Mr. Gizinski, Mr. G we called him, in 5th grade programmed computers with me and expanded my imagination by introducing me to science fiction. Mr. Cornelius taught me the value of right thought, and fairness. And a love of philosophy. I am grateful to both of them for teaching me how we can impact another person's life for the better just by sharing who we are and things we love to do.

And now I am surrounded by amazing people in my life that have helped shape my work and philosophy on helping people.

Cal Banyan is one of the best teachers I have ever had the pleasure of learning from. He taught me more about hypnosis and how the mind works than anyone else on the planet. The motto for his work is "Hypnosis You Can Believe In"™, and it's true. The hypnosis he teaches, and that I use, has worked for hundreds of my clients, and for my student's clients as well. But the amazing thing about Cal is that he's the real deal - he's genuine. Every day I'm grateful for what Cal has taught me about feelings, how the mind works, and how to transform clients into the best versions of themselves. I'm also grateful that he created 7th Path Self-Hypnosis ® which I use every day to continue my own personal growth.

I am grateful for Maureen Banyan because she taught me how to run my business. What I didn't realize when I started my hypnosis business was that the more effectively you run your practice, the more people you can help. I am thankful that Maureen understands the balance between wanting to help people out of the goodness in your heart and the need to do it in a way that also makes business sense so your practice is sustainable.

I am grateful to all of my compassionate colleagues and teachers - Brenda Titus, Karen Hand, Celeste Hackett, Donna Bloom, Laney Coulter, Marcella Hilferty, Kelley Woods, Catherine Johns, Melissa Tiers, Alanna Jackson, and 5-PATH® and HOPE Coaching hypnotists worldwide who help me become a better hypnotist every day through sharing their own work, love, and support. They all taught me the value of surrounding yourself with a diverse collection of talented and compassionate people to help you learn and grow.

Thank you ToiAnn for your relentless support of my work including writing this book and all of our lunchtime talks about change work that helped to shape what I do. Thank you also for introducing me to Difference Press.

Thank you Laura Abernathy for everything you've done for me personally and professionally. From our first session where I created my mission statement, to the realization of my dreams including my hypnosis practice, becoming a hypnosis trainer and paid speaker, and now to writing this book.

There are a few people who, without them this book probably never would have happened. They are my sisters, my close family, and my publishing team.

Thank you Cherish for reviewing this manuscript so many times, for helping me brainstorm ways to say what I want to say in a way that other people can understand. For helping to smooth over all my writing, and dropping down into that very deep, heart-center feeling place with me. I knew that you understood what I was trying to do with this book, and because of that I felt the freedom to create it in a way where I believe my authentic voice was heard.

Thank you Holly, you've inspired my work and writing from the very beginning – since I was 2 and you were moments old. I'm grateful that you saved me on that day that seems so long ago, and now for the various walks in the woods where we share and talk which helps expand my understanding of how to help people and the work I want to do.

Thank you Lindsey, because just by being you, you taught me how to be alive. To be authentic and feel and love every moment of the day.

And for Paige who has always believed in me, and supported me more than anyone else, asking the right questions, and always being there.

This book would not be what it is now without the help and guidance of my publisher – Difference Press, Angela Lauria and my editor Cynthia Kane. I knew the moment I understood the philosophy of Difference Press – books that make a difference, that it was right for me and my message. They taught me how to take my message and make it accessible to readers. How to take what I know, and turn it into something that can be shared in a written format. I learned the value of first understanding who I'm writing the book for, then to return to that place and ensure the message in my book is always on track with my original intention. I learned writing is about continual self-discovery that gets folded back into the message to enrich the value and understanding for the reader. I am grateful that you helped me take my book from an idea to a finished product, and helped me to understand the value of each step along the way.

Very importantly, thank you to all my clients who I learn from every single day.

And thank you to all the readers for trusting in me to help you with your journey. I hope this book has been helpful for you and look forward to hearing from you about your experience reading it and the ways that it helped transform your life.

Each of you have taught me something very important, and I appreciate and value that. And I know I will continue to learn and grow from you, and others, each and every day.

To the Morgan James Publishing team, David Hancock, CEO & Founder, thank you for creating an empowering process for printing this book, and to Megan Malone, Managing Editor, thanks for helping along the way and making the process seamless and easy. To everyone else, Jim Howard, Bethany Marshall, Nickcole Watkins, thanks to each of you for your expertise in helping to guide this book into the hands of people who can benefit from it.

ABOUT THE AUTHOR

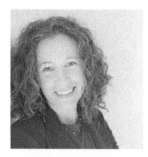

Erika Flint is an award-winning hypnotist, author, speaker, and a co-host of the popular podcast series *Hypnosis, Etc.* She is the founder of Cascade Hypnosis Center in Bellingham, WA, and the creator of the **Reprogram Your Weight** system.

Before becoming a hypnotist, Erika designed software for the high-tech industry. She was working in that field for over a decade when she realized how interested she was in the most powerful computing device available – the human mind. Now she combines her analytical expertise along with powerful hypnosis techniques and her compassion for people to help clients utilize their most powerful asset – their mind.

She has assisted hundreds of clients with weight loss by helping them reprogram how they think and feel. Her unique design and approach helps clients tap into their own inherent power and keep the weight off once and for all.

Erika's heartfelt approach is the trademark of her work. She values authentic connections with people and works to reveal the wonderment at the core of each individual.

She lives in Bellingham, WA with her family including three sweet cats and a happy rescue dog who loves to play soccer.

THANK YOU

Thank you for reading this book. It's my great honor and pleasure to share these ideas with you.

If you're ready to reprogram your weight take the quiz **Can You Reprogram Your Weight?** This short quiz is located online at: ReprogramYourWeight.com/quiz and comes with a free Reprogram Your Weight Toolkit to help you in the next steps of your journey.

There is also a companion online class that goes along with the book. You can find more at ReprogramYourWeight.com/course.

If you're ready to get started on your weight loss journey as soon as possible, working one on one with me is the fastest route. You can get started by filling out the online form here: ReprogramYourWeight.com/consultation. Or you can send me an email at erika@CascadeHypnosisCenter.com.

I would love to speak at your event on the ideas in this book, including hypnosis, weight loss, or how each of us has the power within to be successful and make any change we want to in our lives. Visit ReprogramYourWeight.com/speaking for more information or contact me at erika@CascadeHypnosisCenter. com to get started.

I look forward to hearing from you. Until then, be well and know that someone (me) cares about you and your well-being.

With much love,

Erika

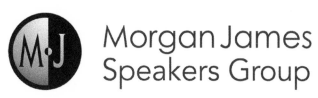

Morgan James
Speakers Group

www.TheMorganJamesSpeakersGroup.com

We connect Morgan James published
authors with live and online events
and audiences whom will benefit
from their expertise.

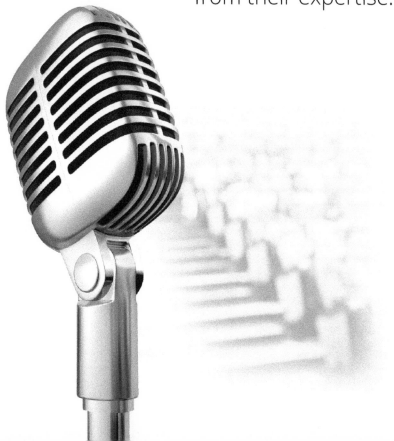

9 781683 502869